A HEART WARRIOR BLOOMS

Written by Ashley K. George

Illustrated by Sara Abbas

A Heart Warrior Blooms
Copyright © 2024 by Ashley K. George

Published in the United States by Elli Twy Kids,
an imprint of Elli Twy Publishing, New York.
www.ellitwy.com

Printed in the United States
First Edition: February 2024

All rights reserved. No portion of this book may be reproduced in any form without permission from the publisher, except as permitted by United States copyright law.

Illustrated by Sara Abbas

Book cover and design by Sadie Butterworth-Jones
www.luneviewpublishing.co.uk

For inquiries, contact the publisher via e-mail: **team@ellitwy.com**

ISBN: 979-8-9861216-3-5 [paperback]
ISBN: 979-8-9861216-4-2 [hardcover]

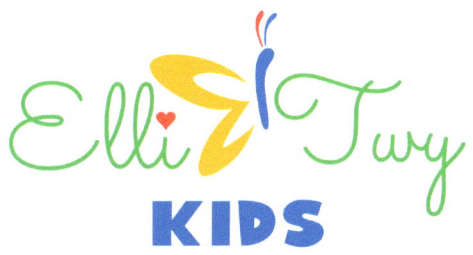

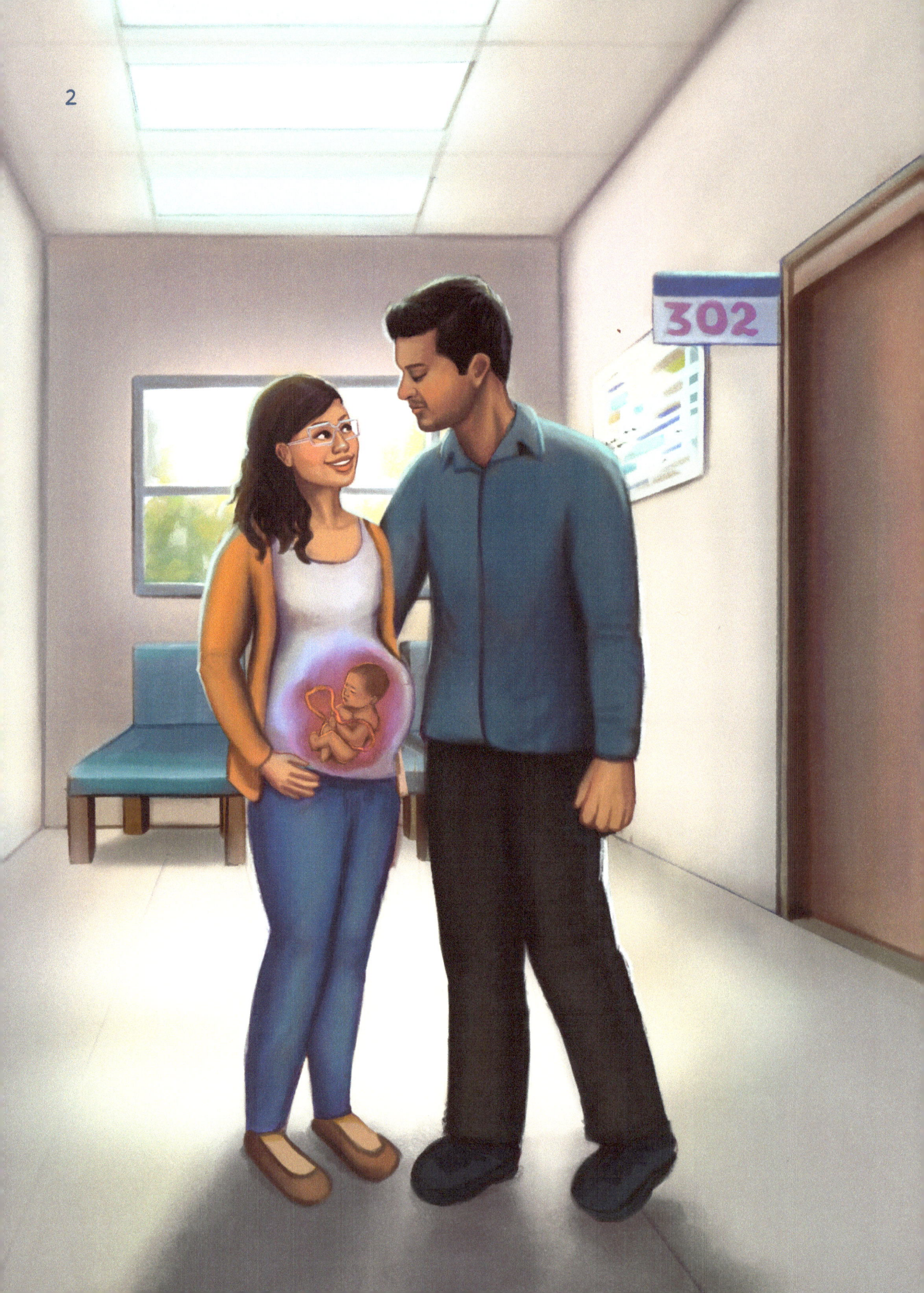

Glimmering, shimmering little hope

eyes closed, thumb in little mouth,

holding onto Mommy's rope

Stifled sighs, happy cries,

joyful tears in parents' eyes

Doctor's office calls them in,

will their little baby win?

Their hearts thump and bump,

pounding voices echo within

The doctor pries,

The doctor spies,

spewing way too many lies,

"You should break these silly ties!"

Mommy cries, Daddy sighs

but baby pushes on and defies

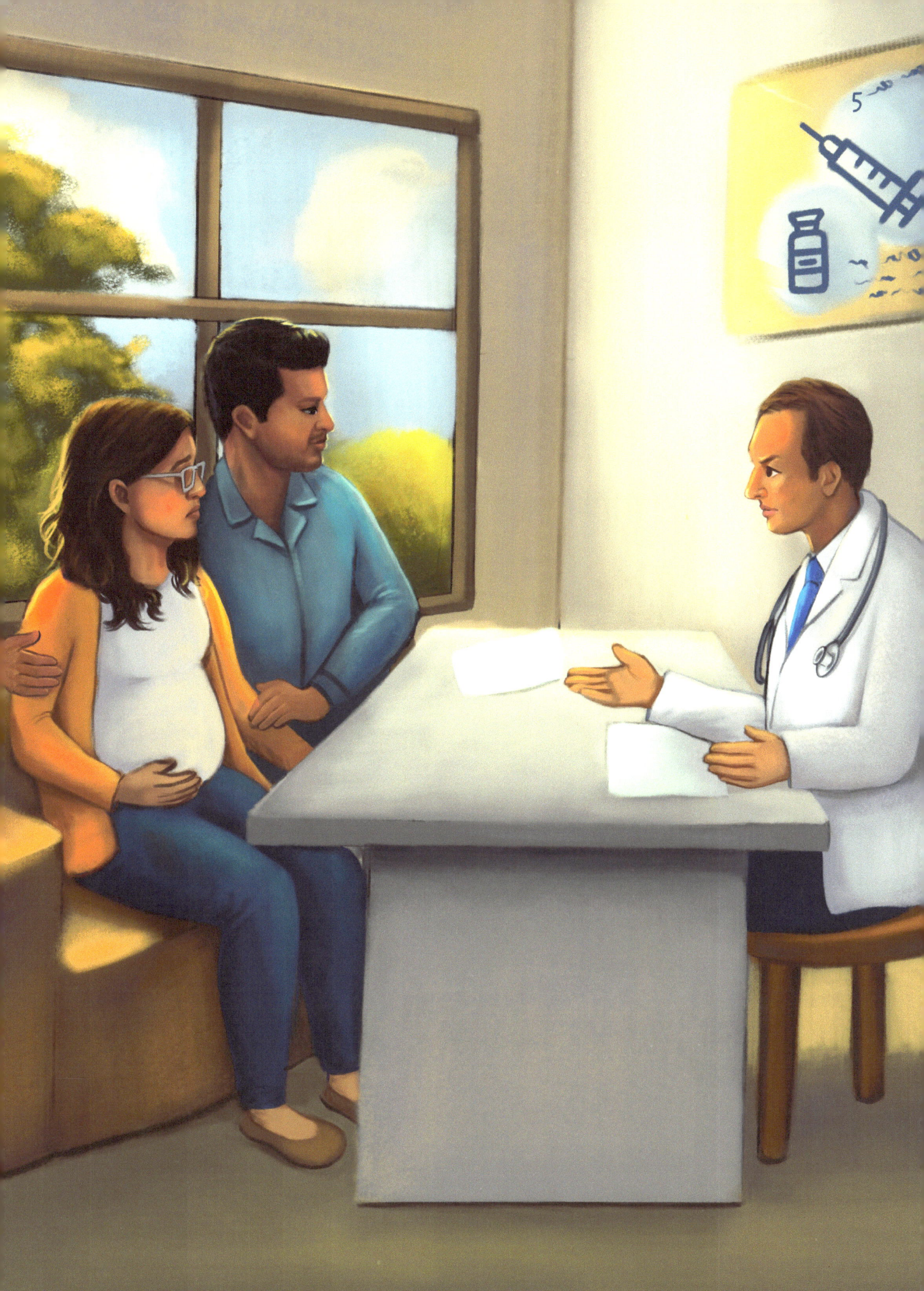

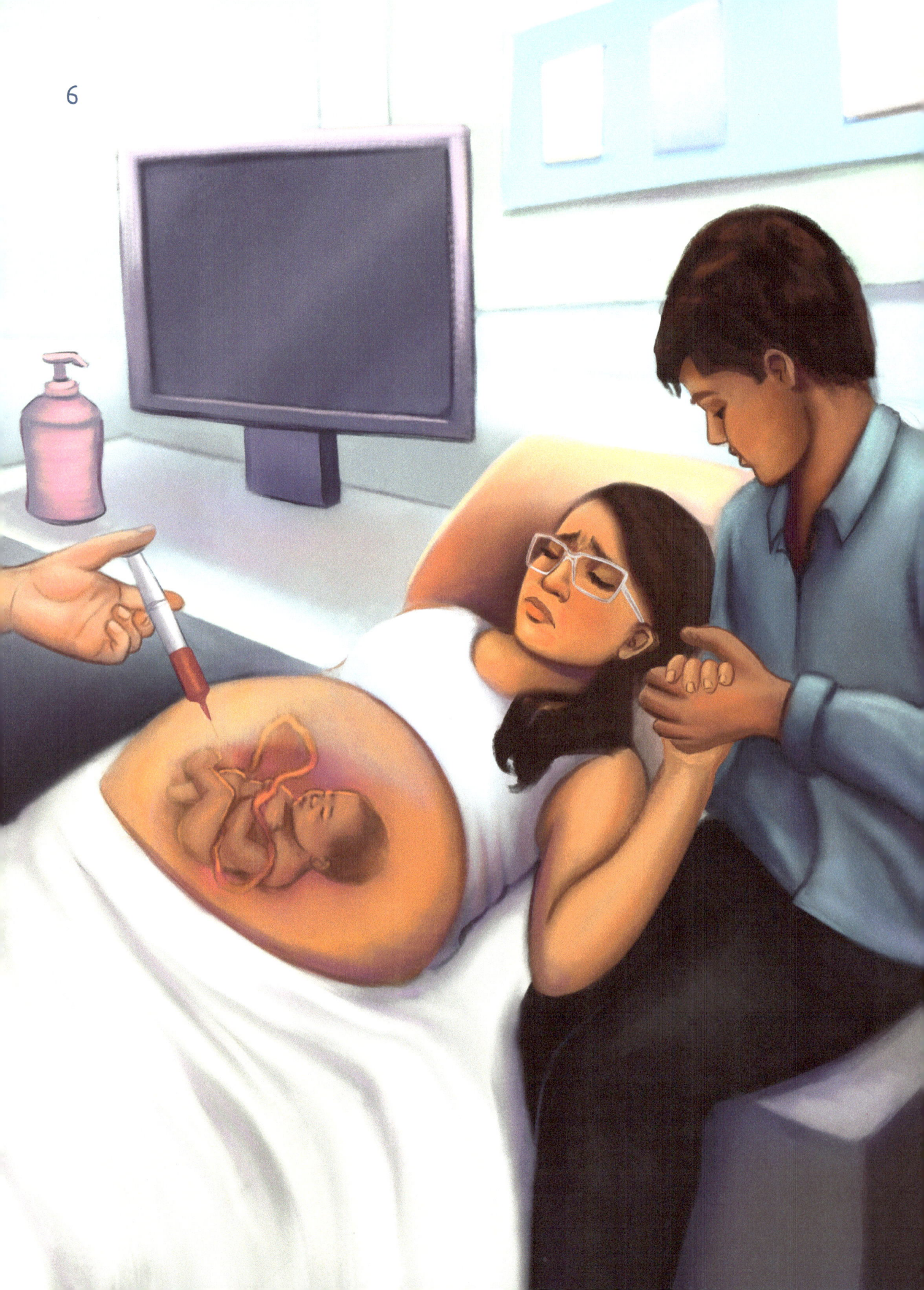

The needle piercing, poking through Mommy, hurts her so BAD

Mommy's sad and Daddy's mad,

there seems no reason to be glad

They say that baby's heart is big on the left side

Yet he flutters happily, drifting in the warm, cozy tide

His eyes closed shut, sleeping, bouncing in his Mommy ride

Baby tosses, kicking happily on Daddy's nose

Mommy picks her favorite red rose,

tickling and caressing her baby's toes

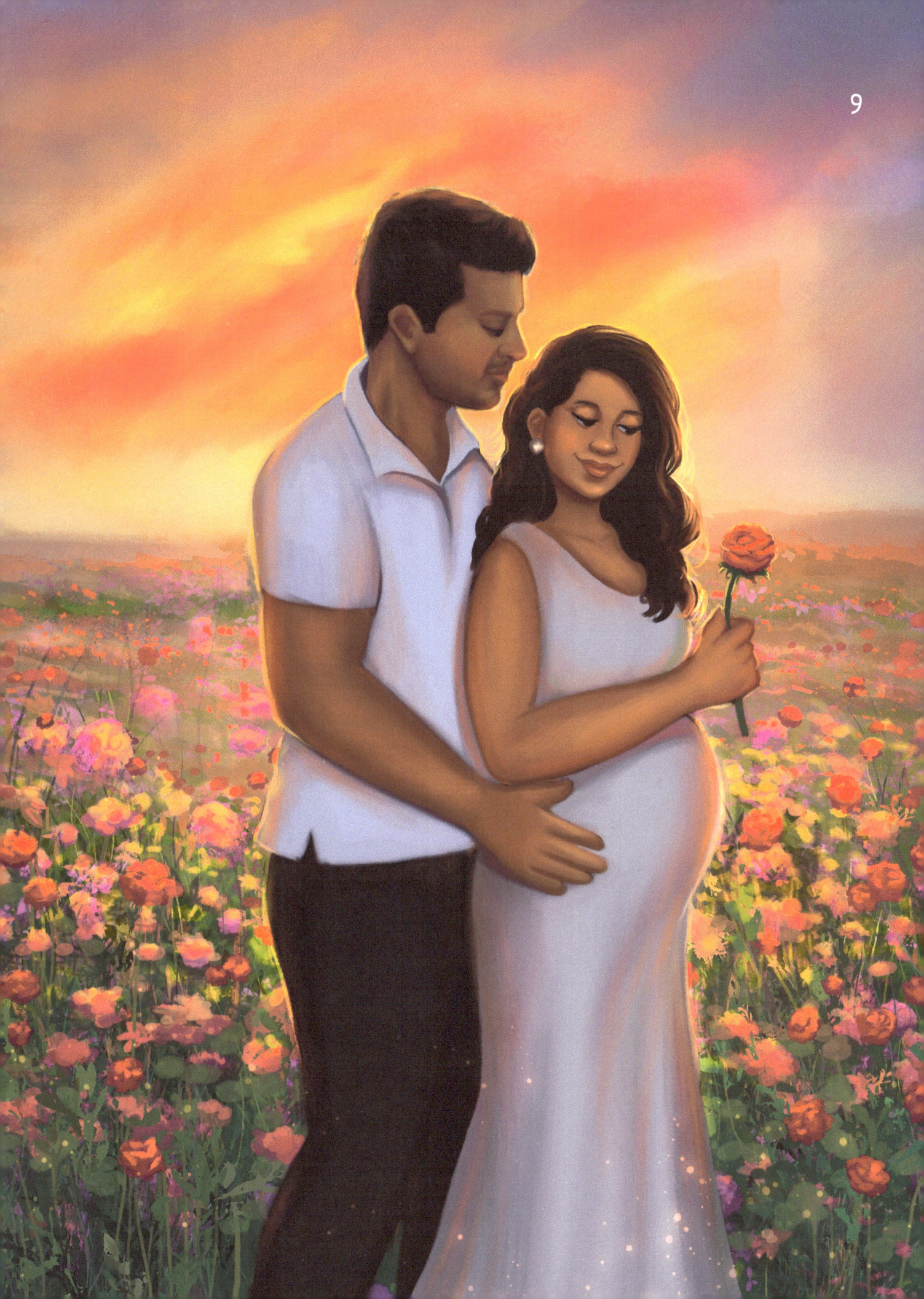

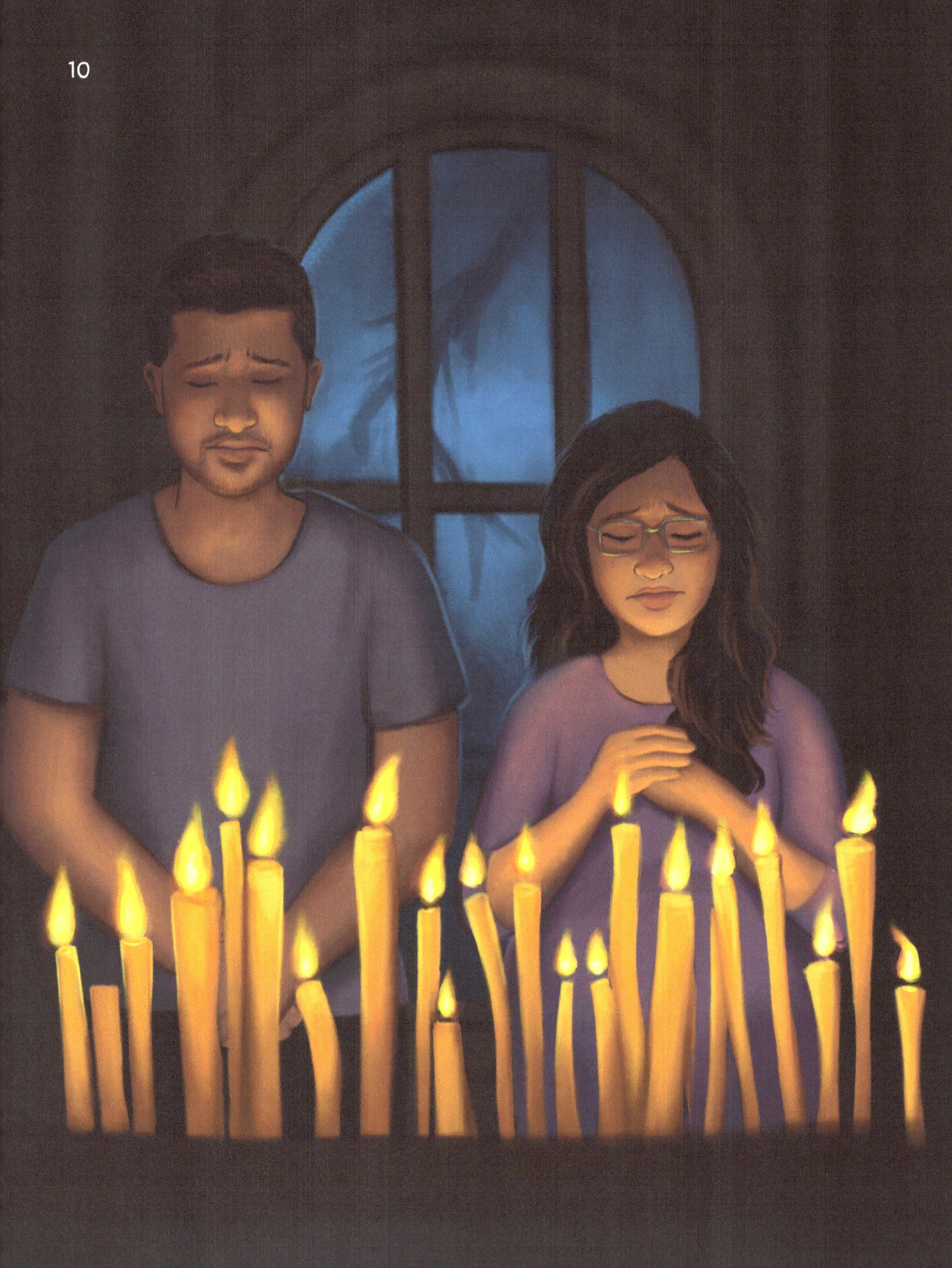

So many scans,

Change of plans,

Baby's heart may have some tear,

but those scans were so unclear

Prayers, whispers, God SPEAKS here,

Bursts of rising hope to appear

Happy cheers, bye bye fear...

"Baby's coming!" exaltations

Almost time for felicitations

Baby's coming, rumbling, tumbling

his heart beat rising, falling, dropping, fumbling

Daddy tightly grasps on to Mommy's hands

As baby pushes into new, unknown lands

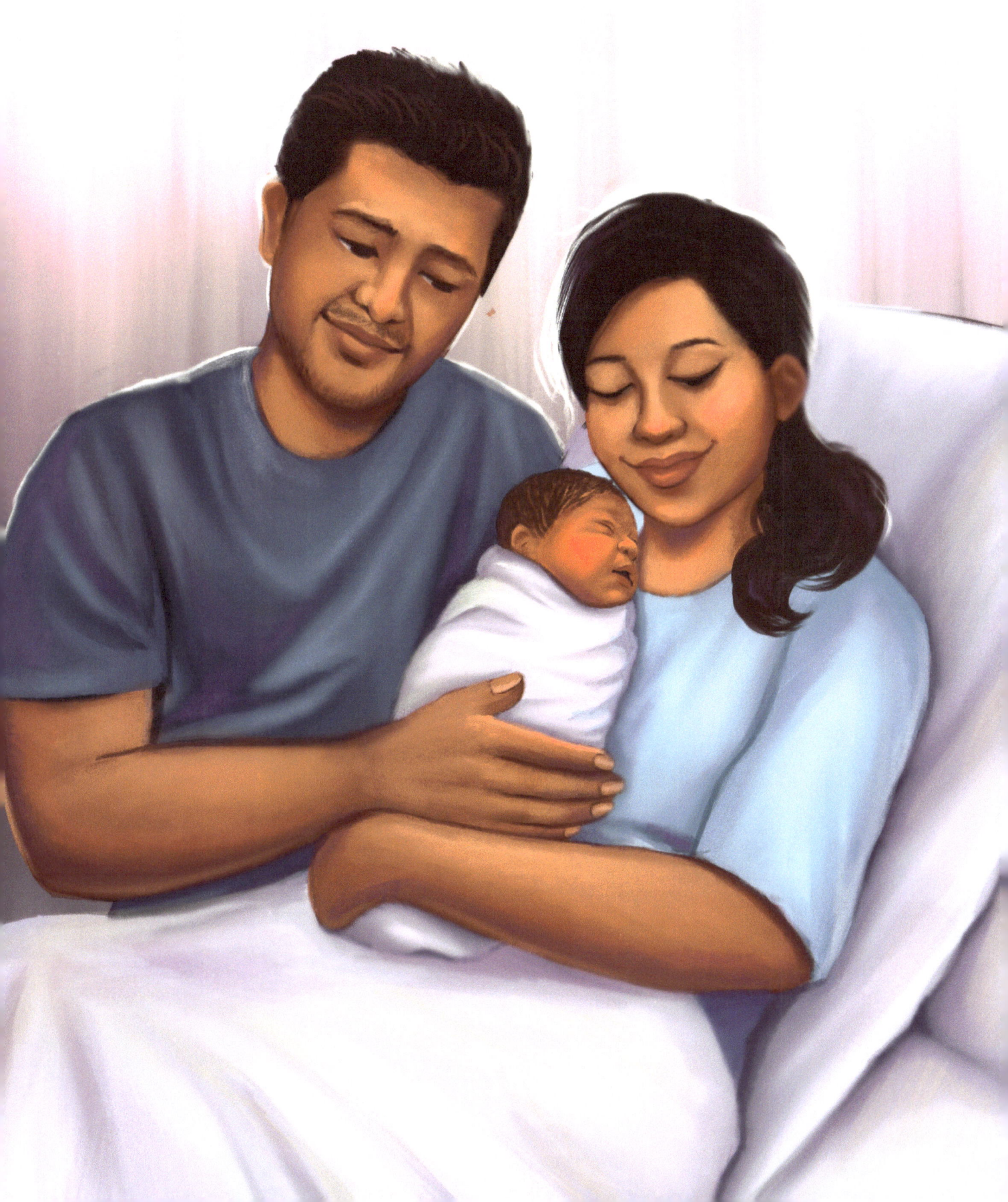

14

Baby's OUT
Looking into his Daddy's eyes,
Whispers quiet sighs,
Smirking, squirming, little POUT

Growing up,

tummy time wiggles,

cherubim inspired giggles

Mommy and Daddy love you dear,

now there seems nothing to fear!

For a while, all is good

and you really seem to like your food

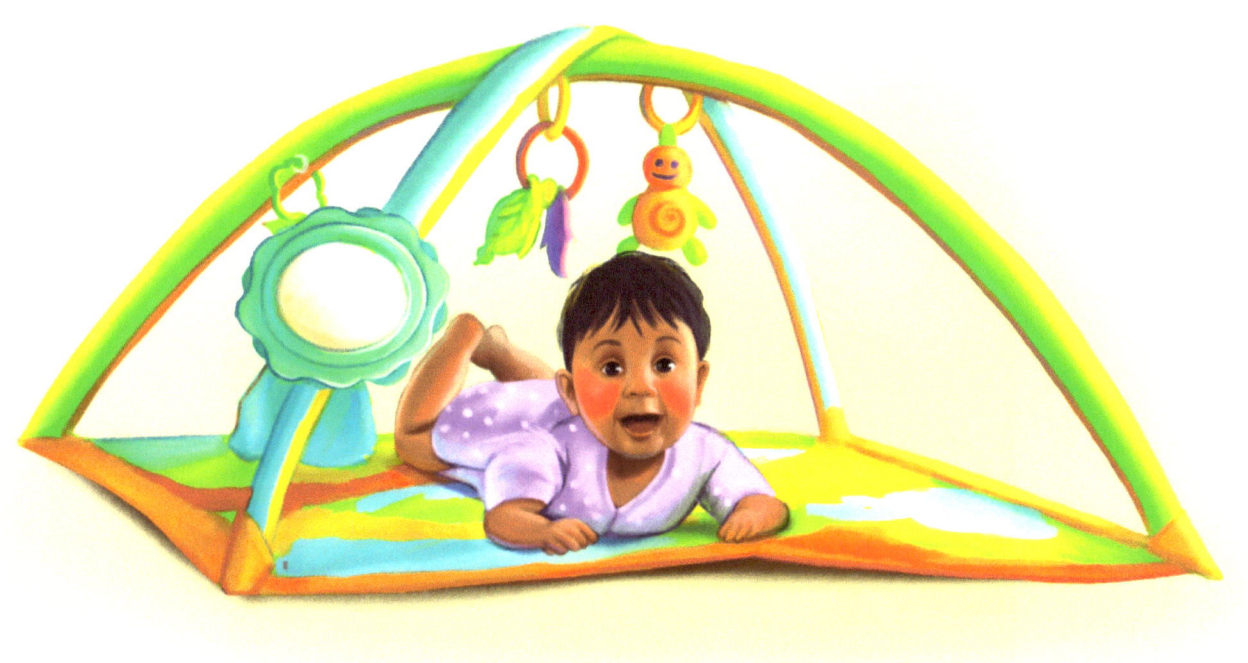
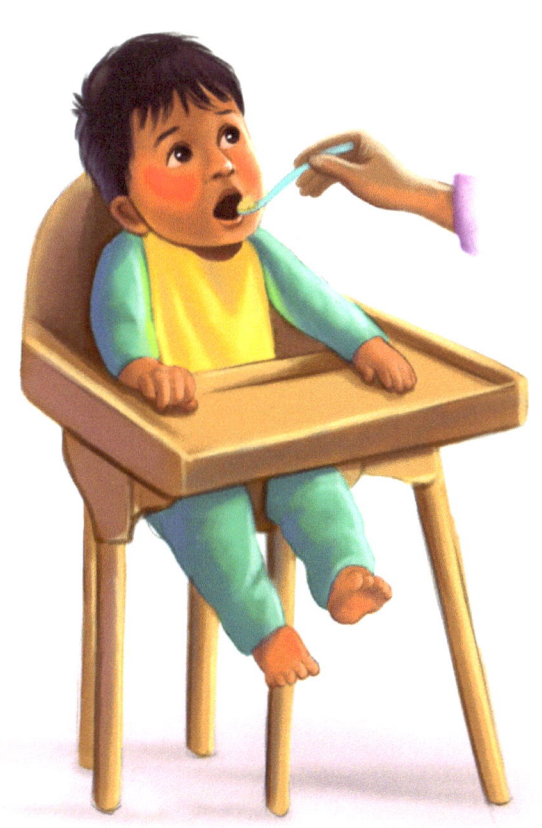

18

As you grow into your nursery,

they learn about your need for surgery

coarctation of the aorta doctors say,

tears crashing, walls closing in on them

On that once happy day

Month 4 baby; they trekked close to a hundred miles away

To dear Uncle's and Aunty's house where they stay,

because there was no other way

That night, all they did was pray

just to see you, and be with YOU another day

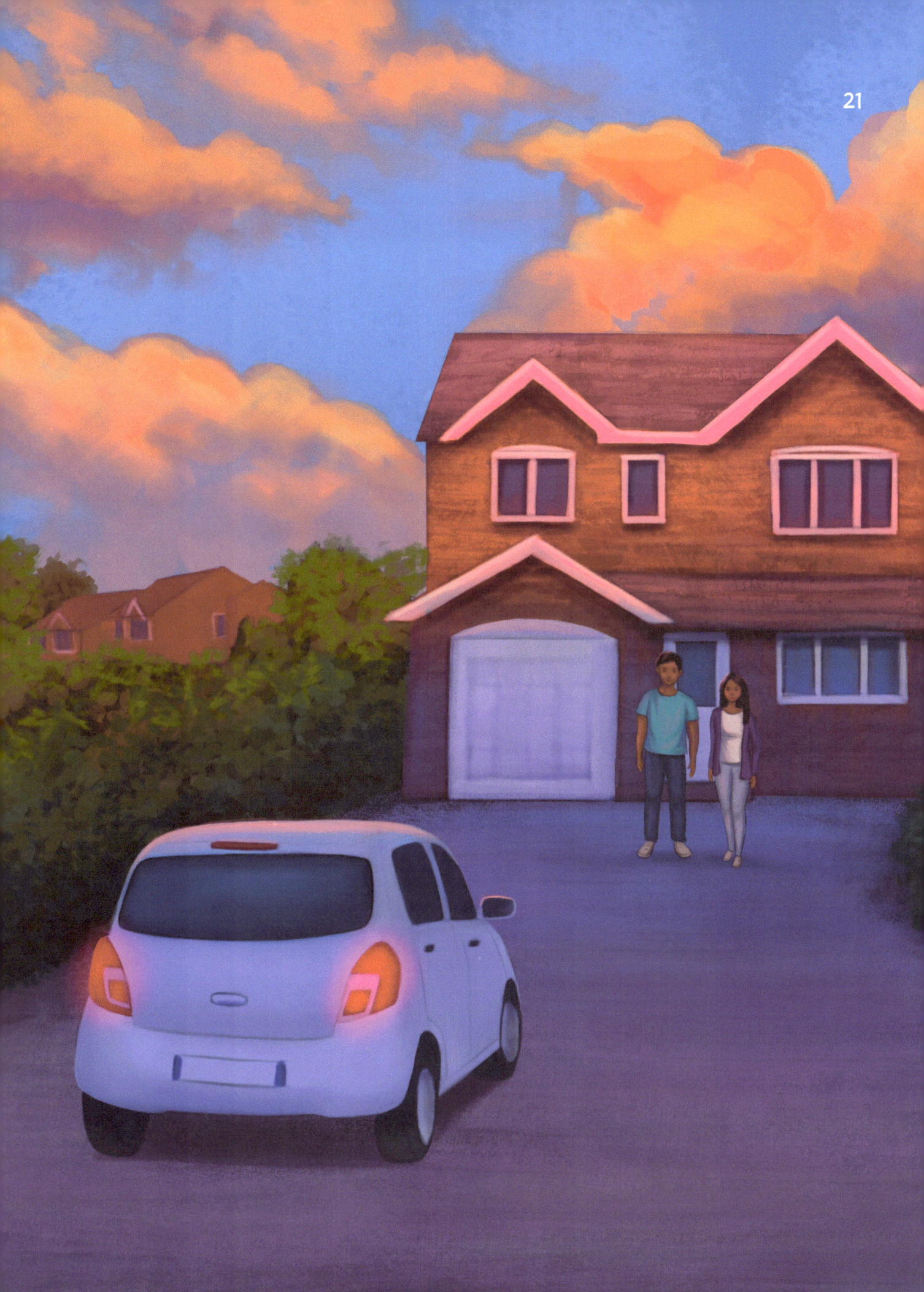

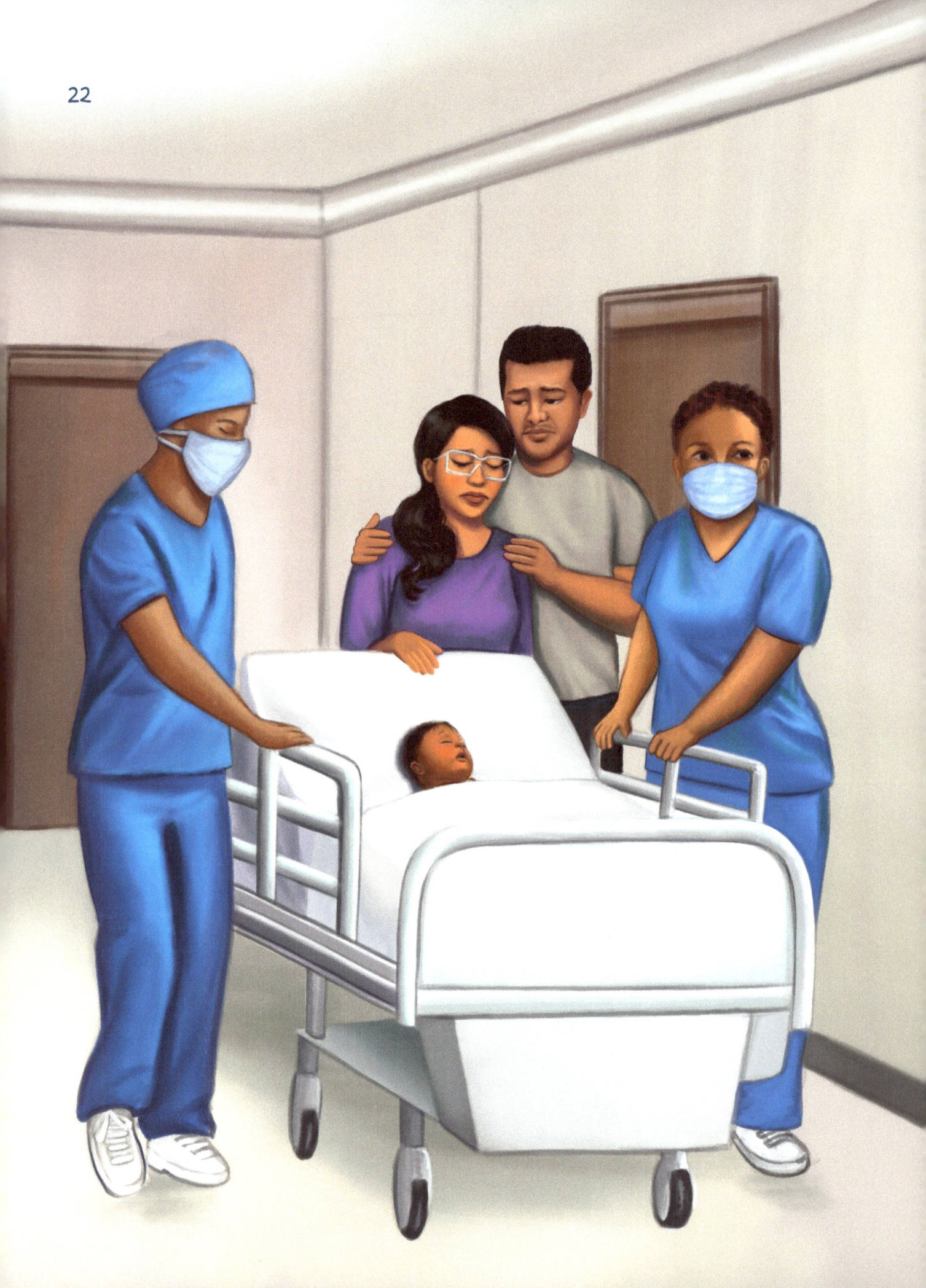

Mommy's hands held you tight as kind nurses carried you away

Daddy held Mommy as she felt her heavy-hearted sway

When her baby was being pulled away

Baby's parents were drenched in pain, tears,

but a rainbow of hope shone on that cloudy day

Baby then became a Heart Warrior,

That coarctation became inferior

Doctors, they stitched it up and closed it tight

Made it right,

For now, no more fright

"Beware" they warned, there is no "cure"

Hazy visions still obscure

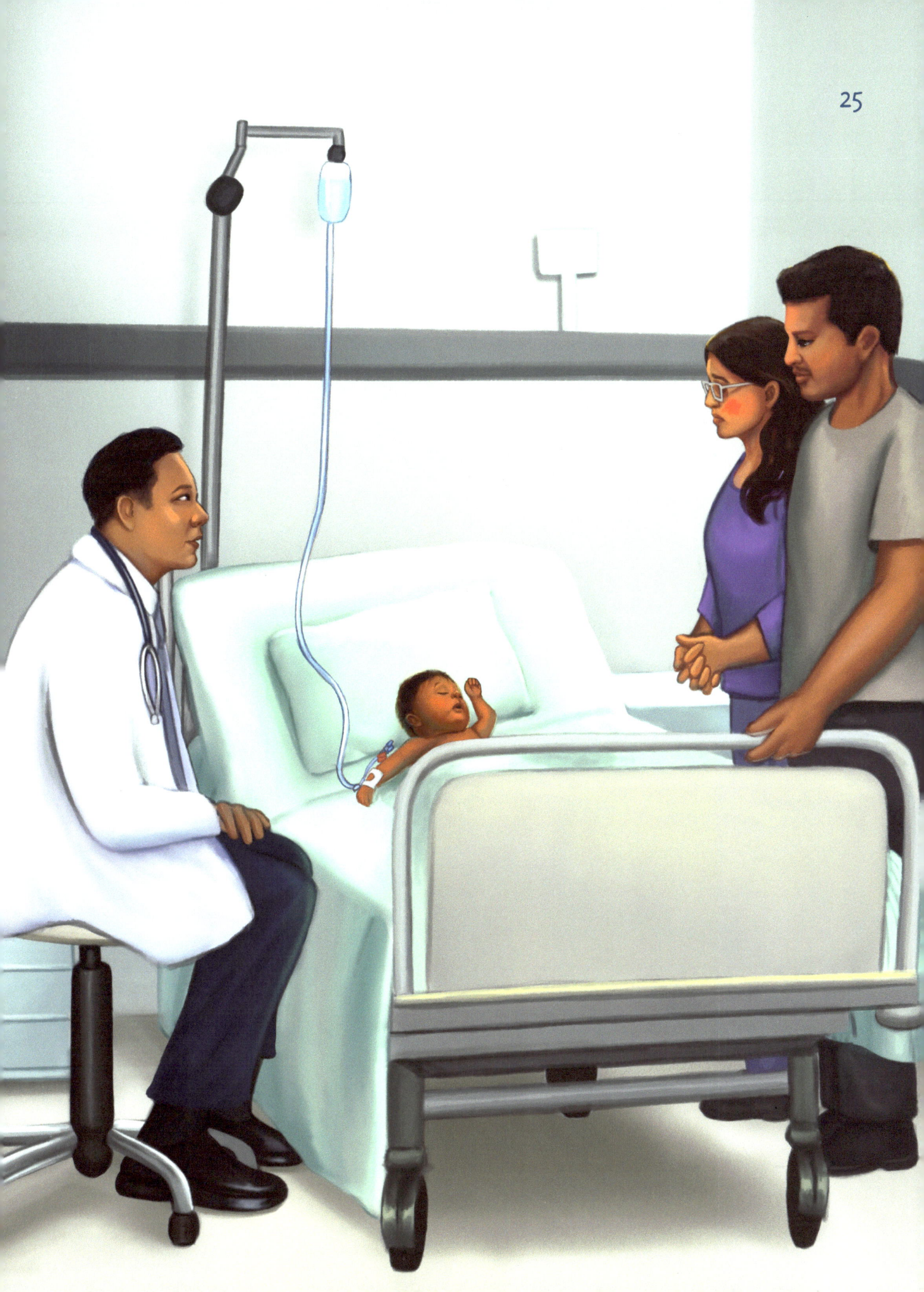

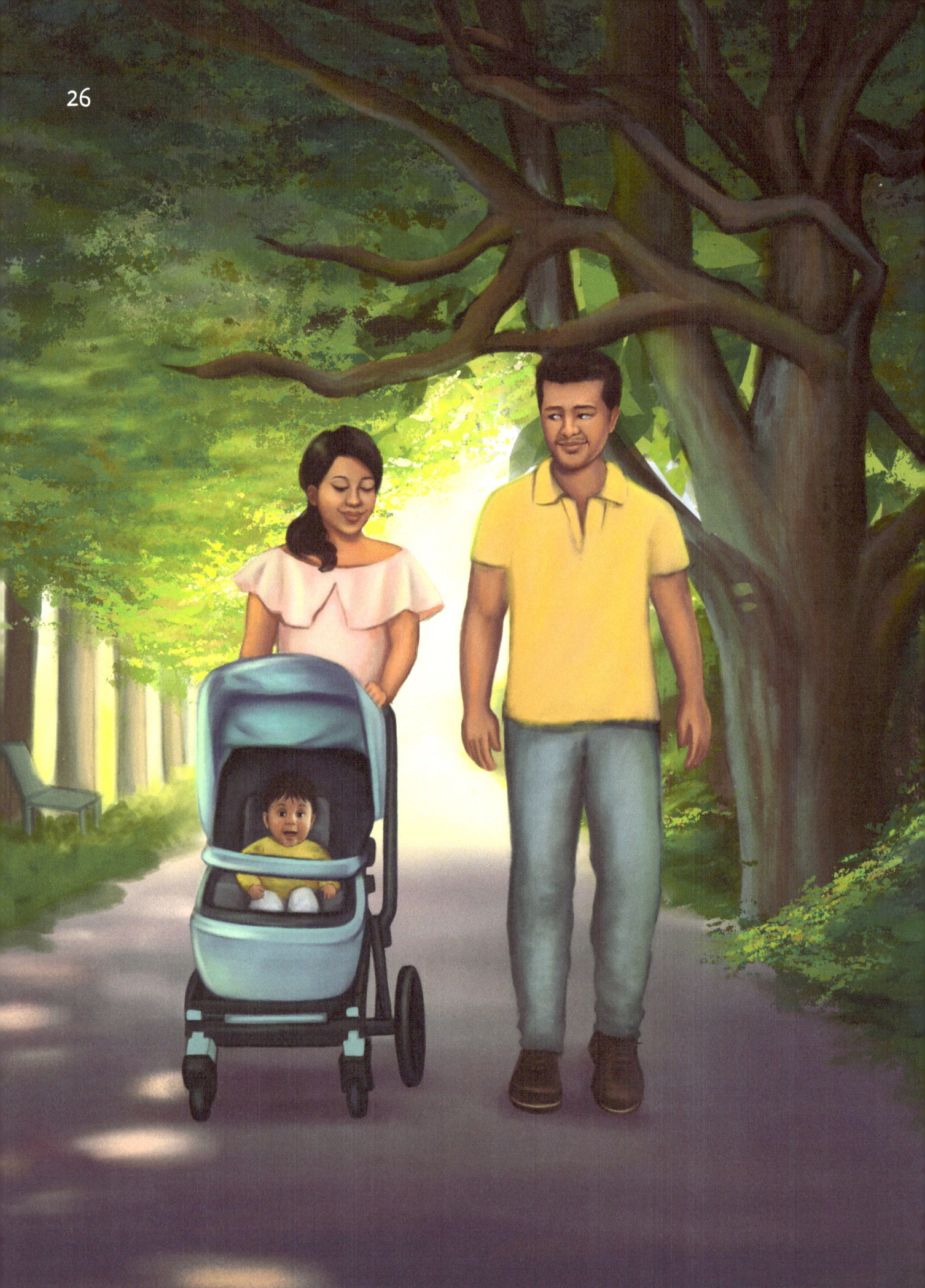

Growing more,

Loving more

his parents hearts became less sore,

baby signed, and baby whined

Baby fed,

baby read,

and baby loved to go to bed

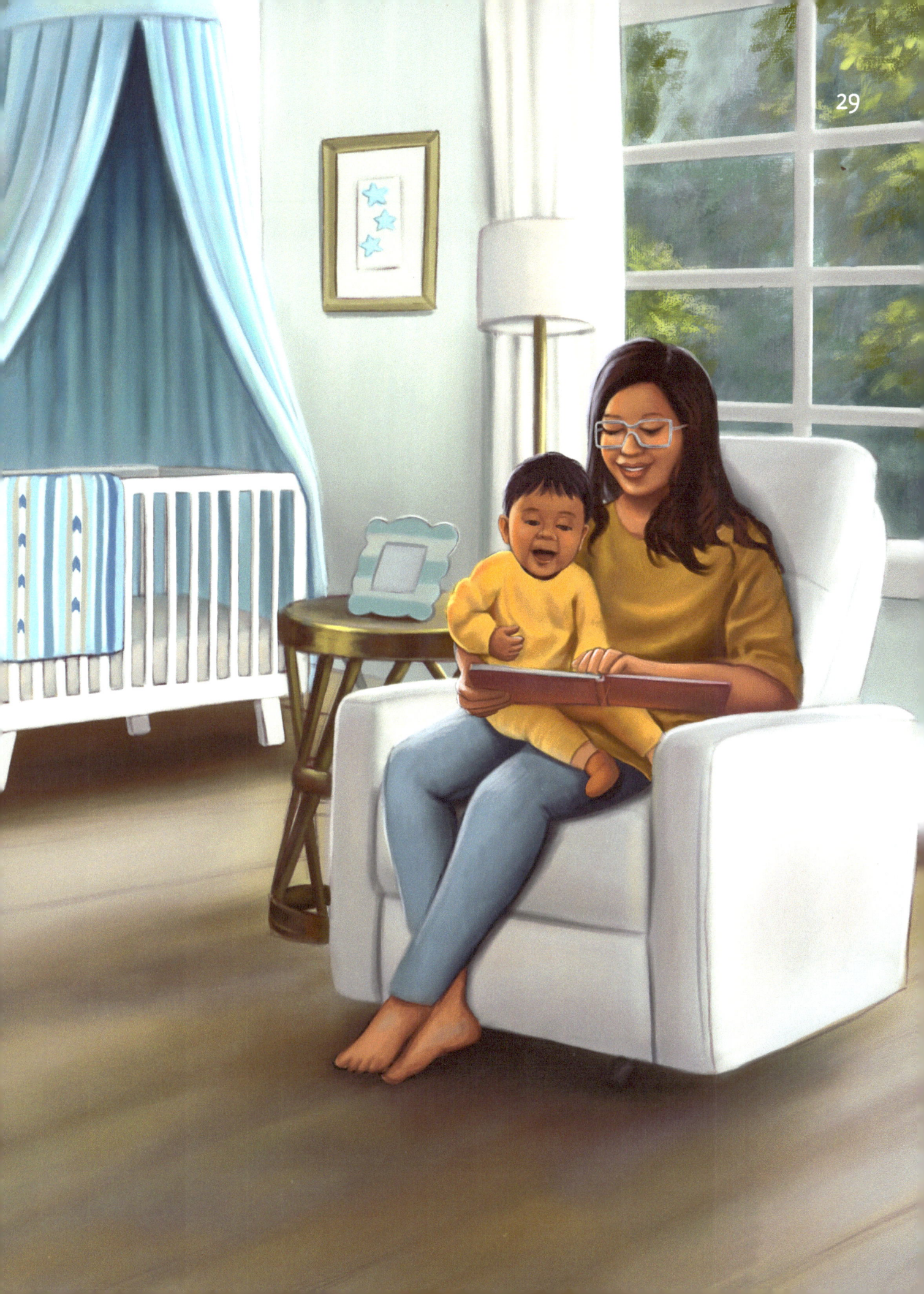

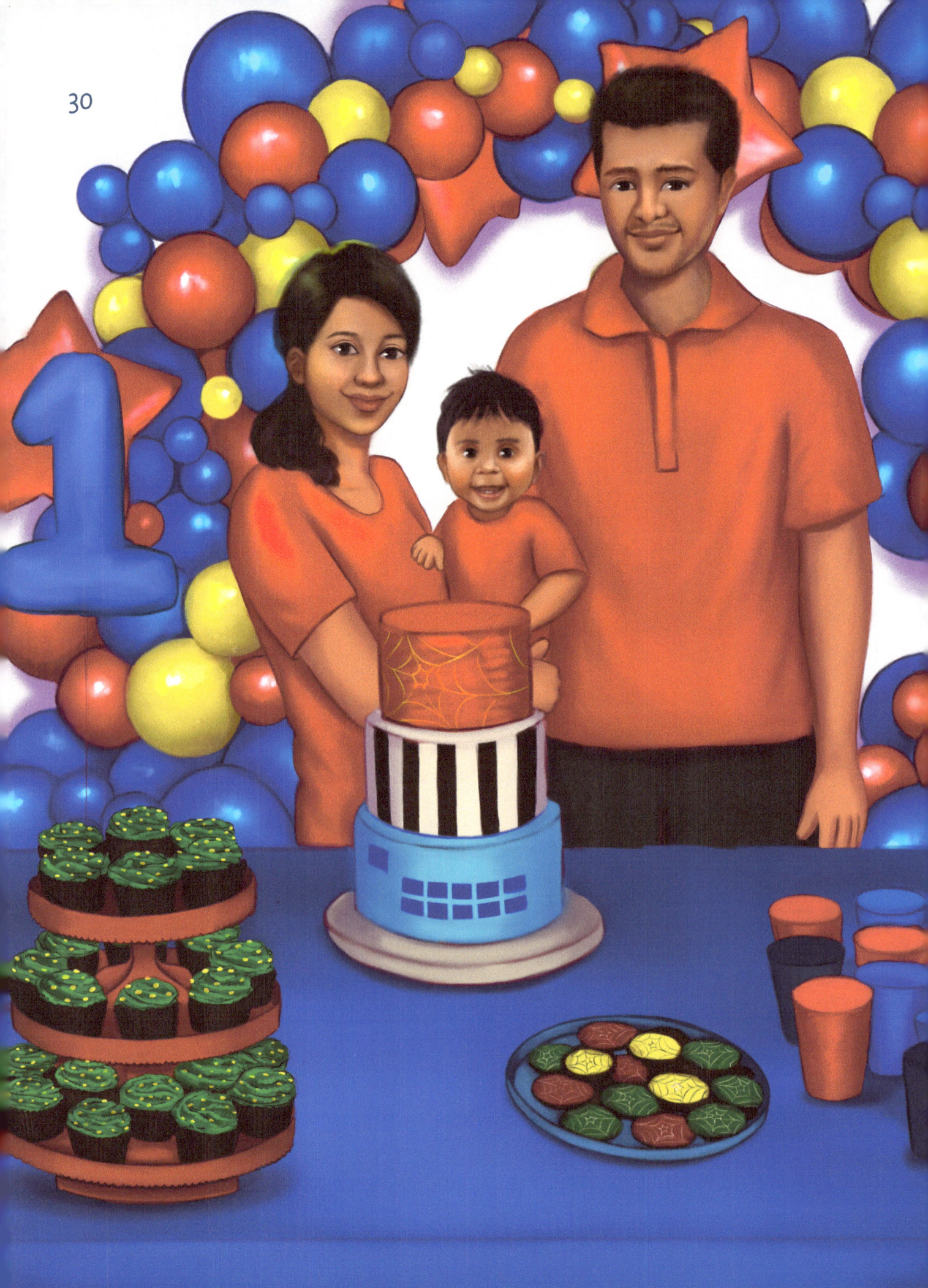

Baby meets more smiling faces,

Pushing through long tummy time races,

Struggling to stand up,

couldn't lift more than a cup

But, with a little help to speed up his pace,

Unhappy, then a happy face

Baby had now found his place

Walking, running, jumping, baby caught up in the race

Baby boy, there are no "delays",

there's always time to work and play,

and grow again another day,

there are stumbles, falls, and pushes that make baby sway

Mommy tells him, "you'll always find another way!"

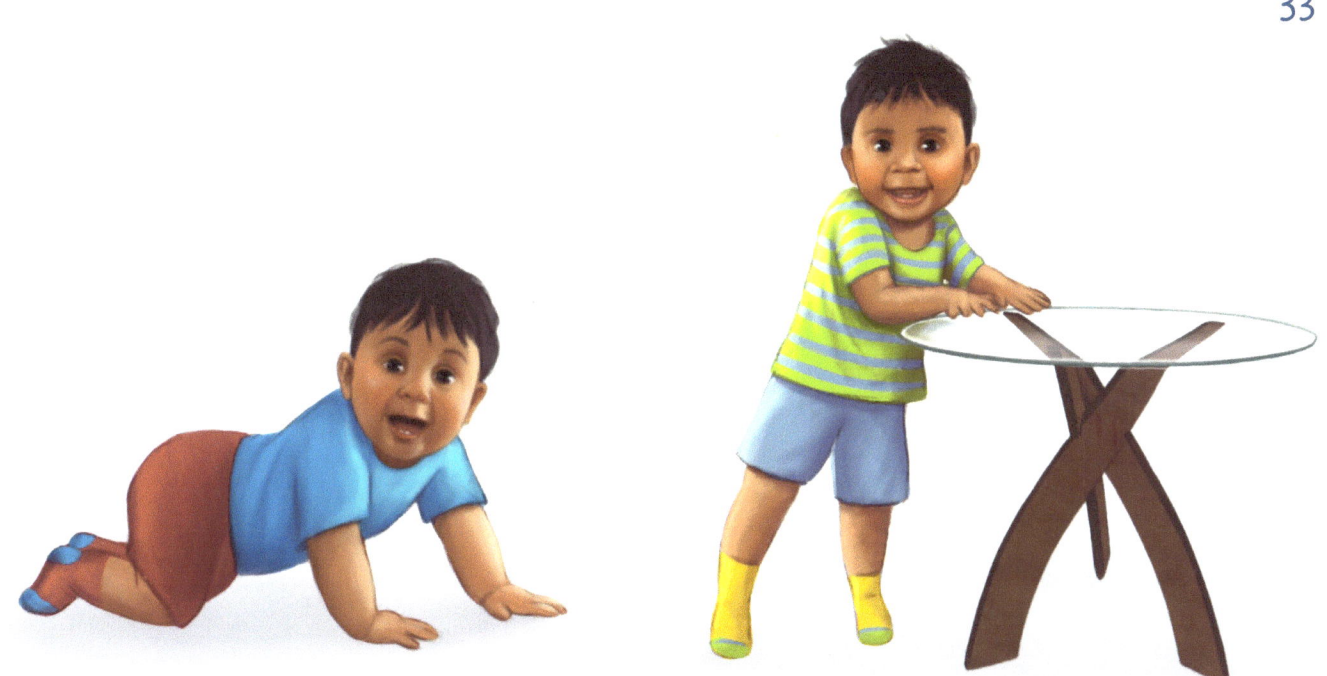

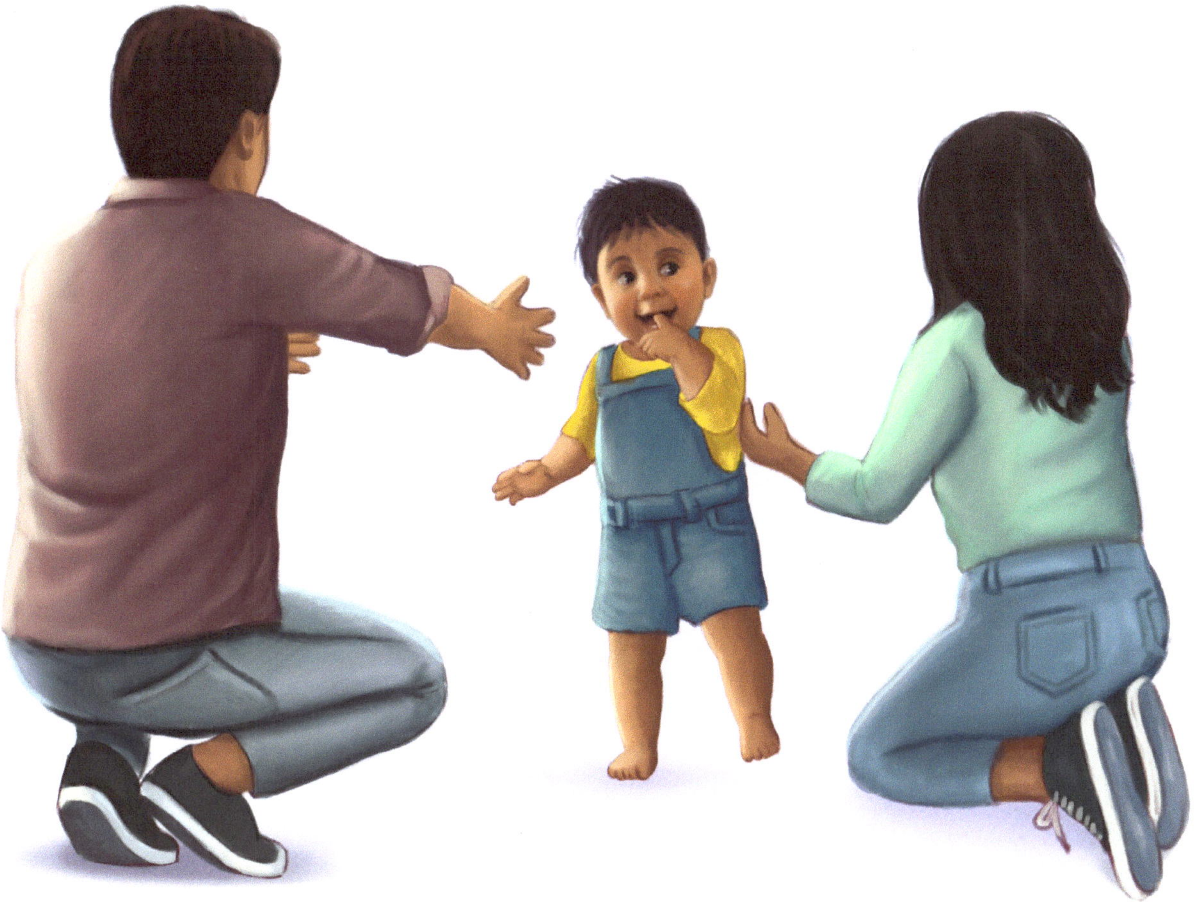

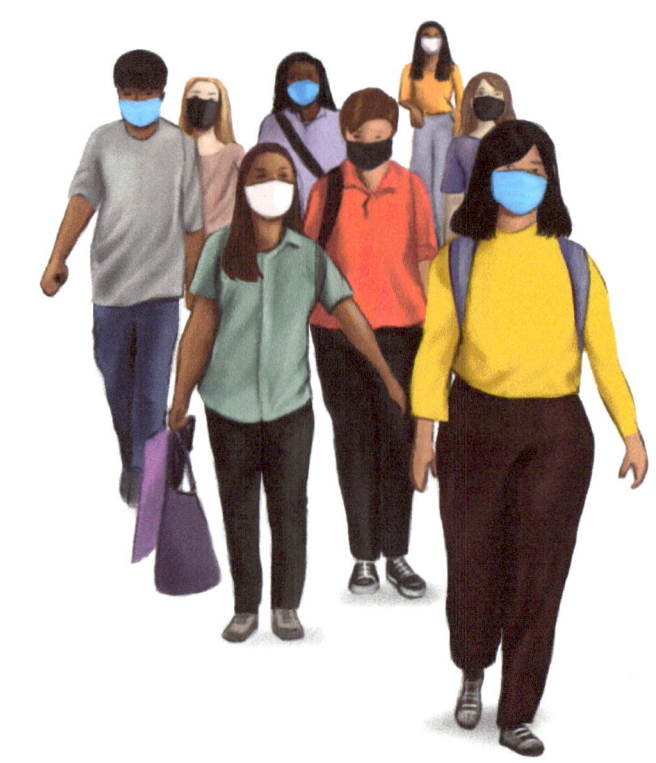
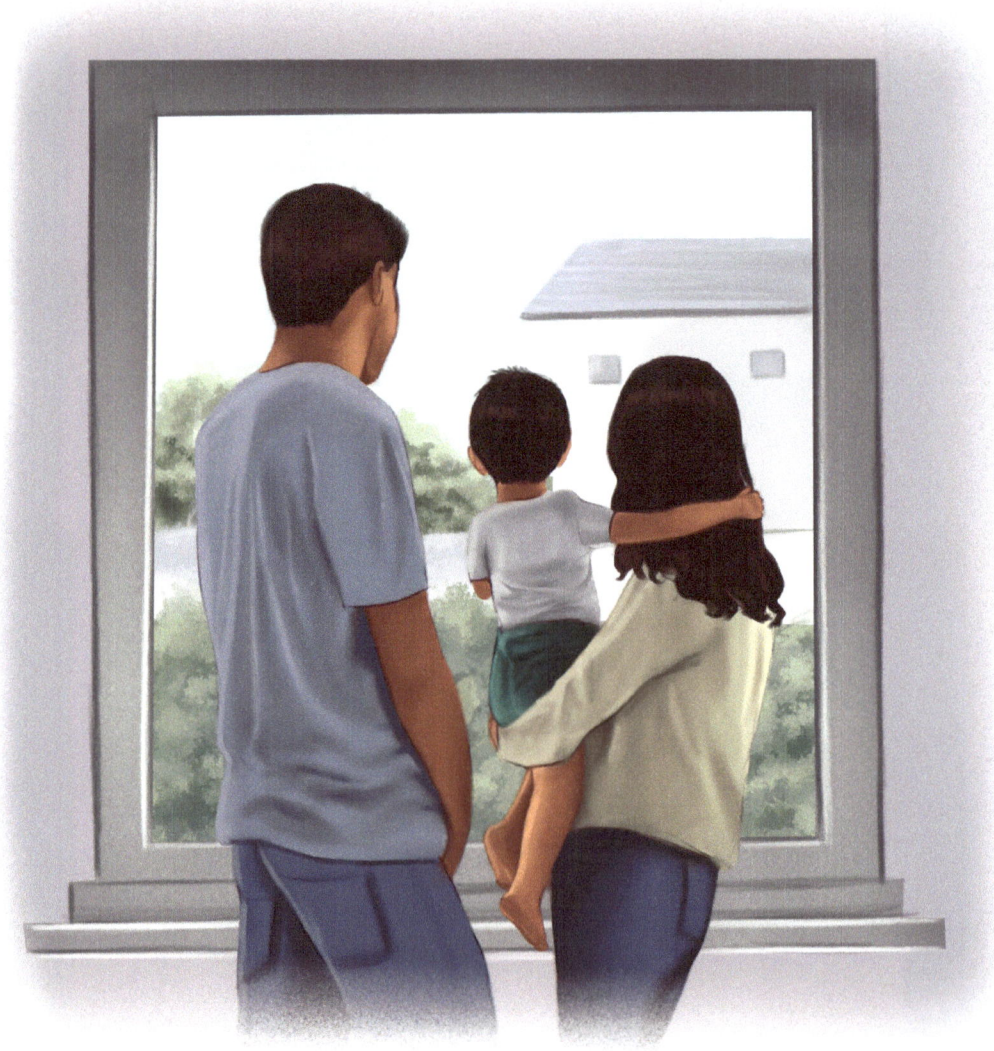

Pandemic paces,

Cloth masked faces,

They navigate through empty places

They must stay home,

There's nowhere to roam

But,

At 2, a newborn sister!

She coos at him with loving whispers,

He teaches her to laugh, smile, running in round loops and twisters

Spinning circles, playing toys,

she follows him; that silly boy

They learn together,

They grow together,

They love together

They fight together,

They laugh together

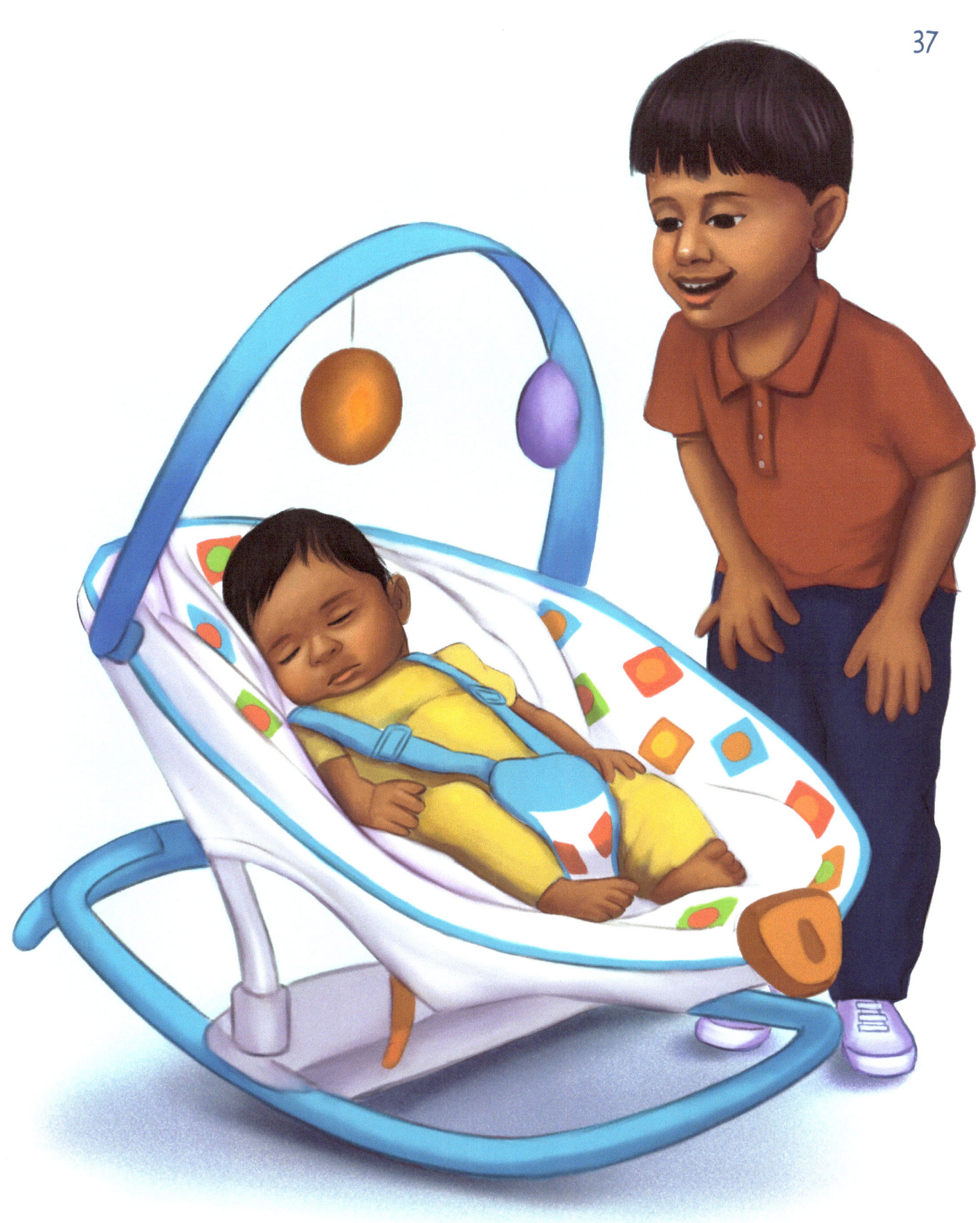

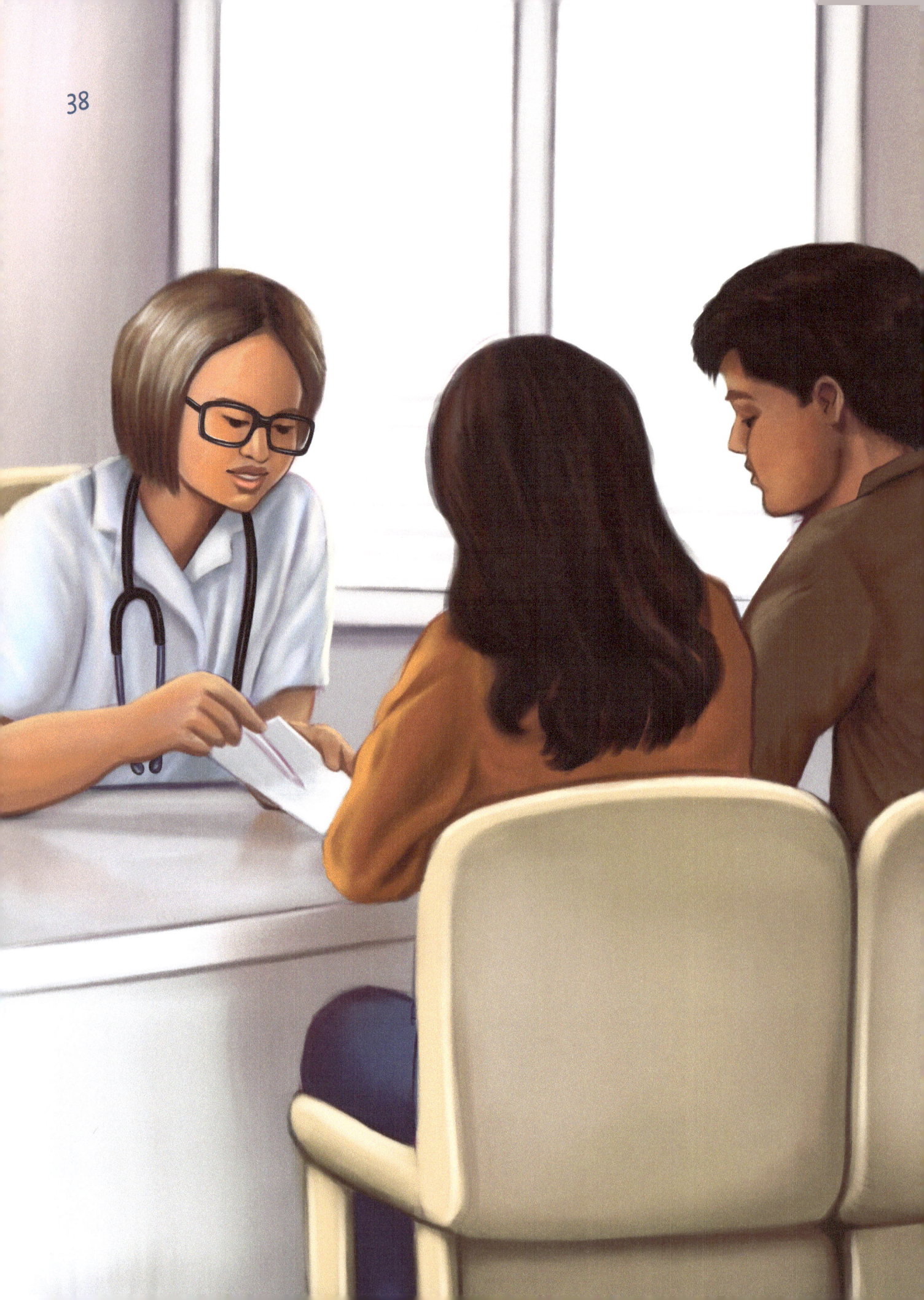

Heart surgery 2 has drawn near
Mommy whimpers out of fear
she cuddles her sweet Boy dear
and wipes away a falling tear

An atrial septal defect and mitral valve cleft
they say; hopefully no other defects left
But, this one too, feels like a theft
and leaves the family feeling bereft

Down goes family's happiness,
Baby sister is put in a dress,
Mommy, Daddy under stress
Baby sister driven to her grandparents' address,
Mommy and Daddy love her always, nonetheless

Gentle kisses on her soft baby head,
A gentle click into her car seat bed,
see you soon our little dear,
Mommy, Daddy, and brother will always be near
So don't you ever have that fear

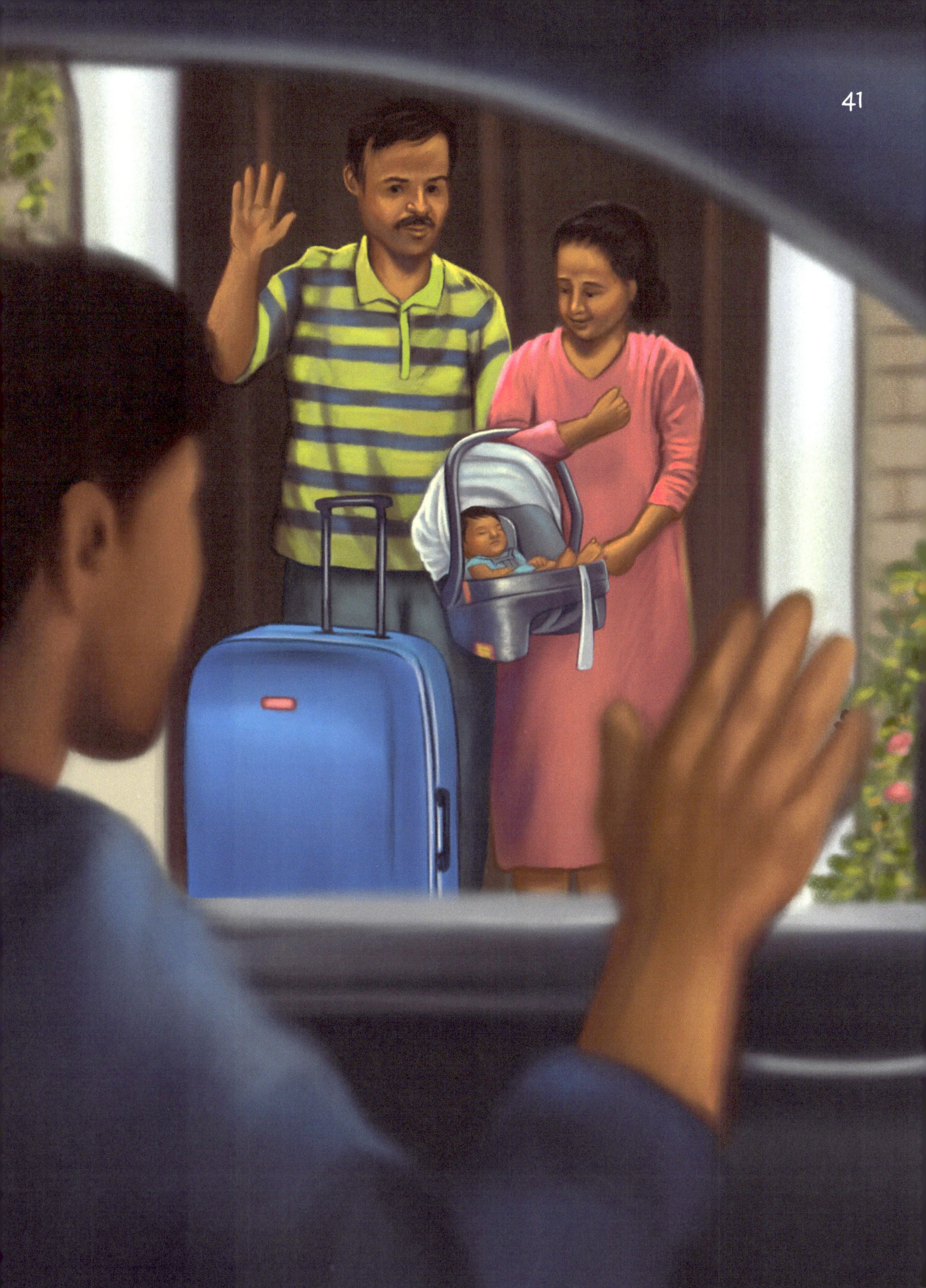

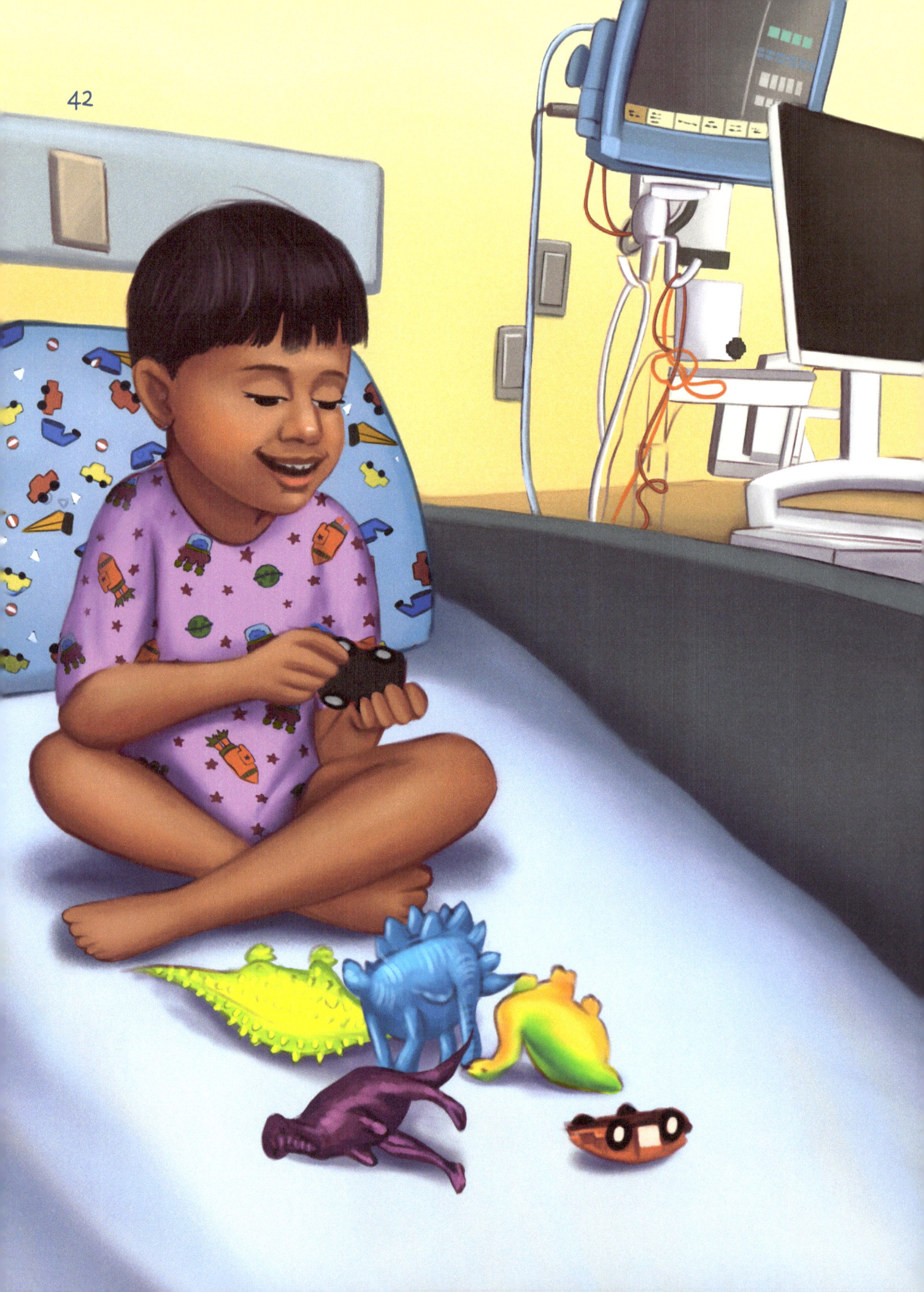

Boy sits with Mommy and Daddy on the hospital bed,

Nurses give him toys to play with before he rests his weary head,

Mommy wishes it were her instead

So many dreams flash in her head

Waiting, waiting – hours pass,

Mommy sips cold water in a glass

Daddy listens to music albums en masse,

Butterflies outside flutter through deep, green grass

Boy's resting in the sleeping gas

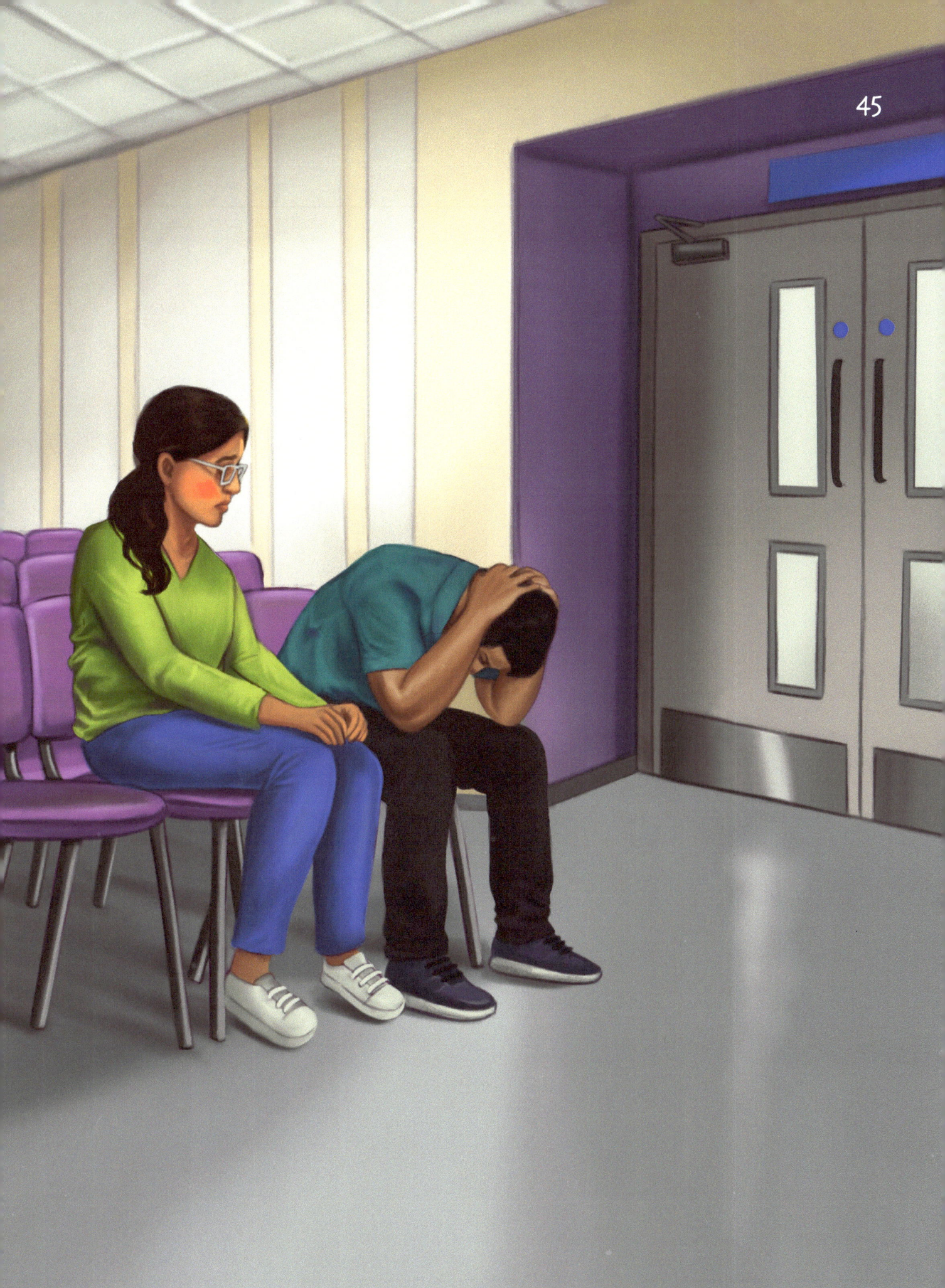

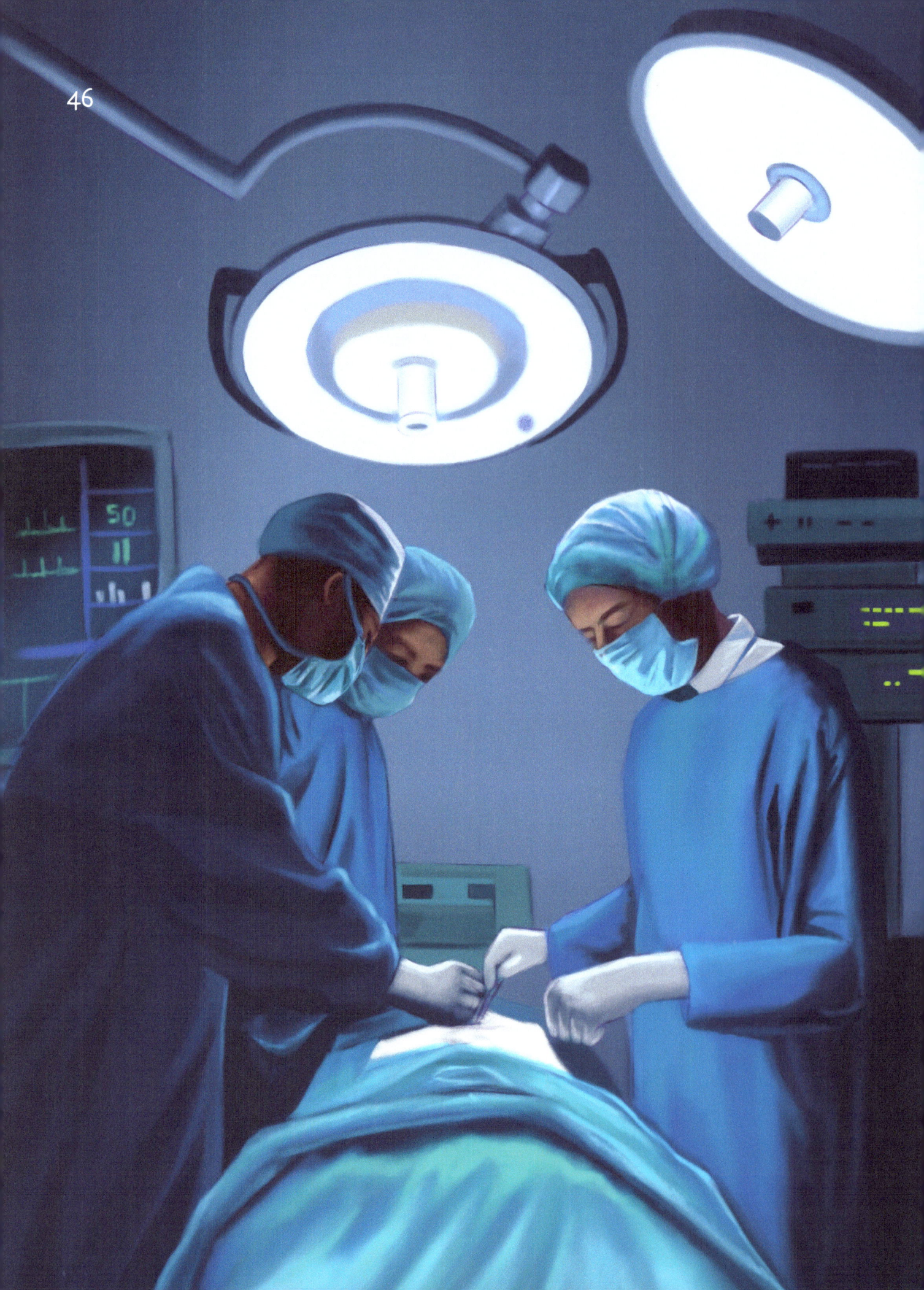

Surgeon stops his little heart,

Several hours before it can restart

Stitching closed holes that once drifted apart

Fixing up his strangely shaped mitral valve defect,

In hope his little body would no longer reject

Because the surgeon knows how to connect

His surgeon: a strong, kind, humble body architect

They wheel him into another room

Surgery's over, no more doom?

Fears and tears constantly loom,

Boy's eyes still closed, Daddy and Mommy's hearts go boom boom

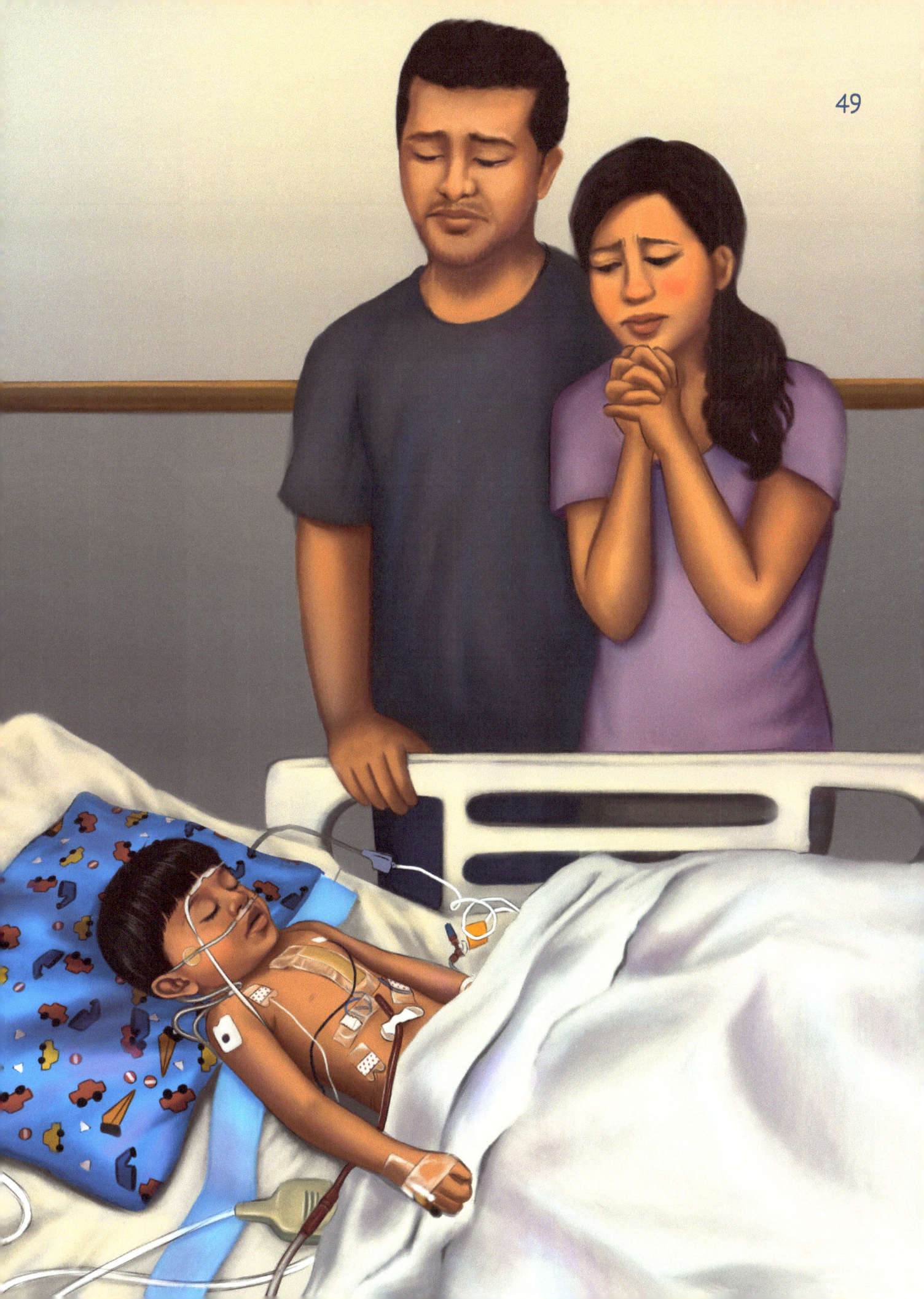

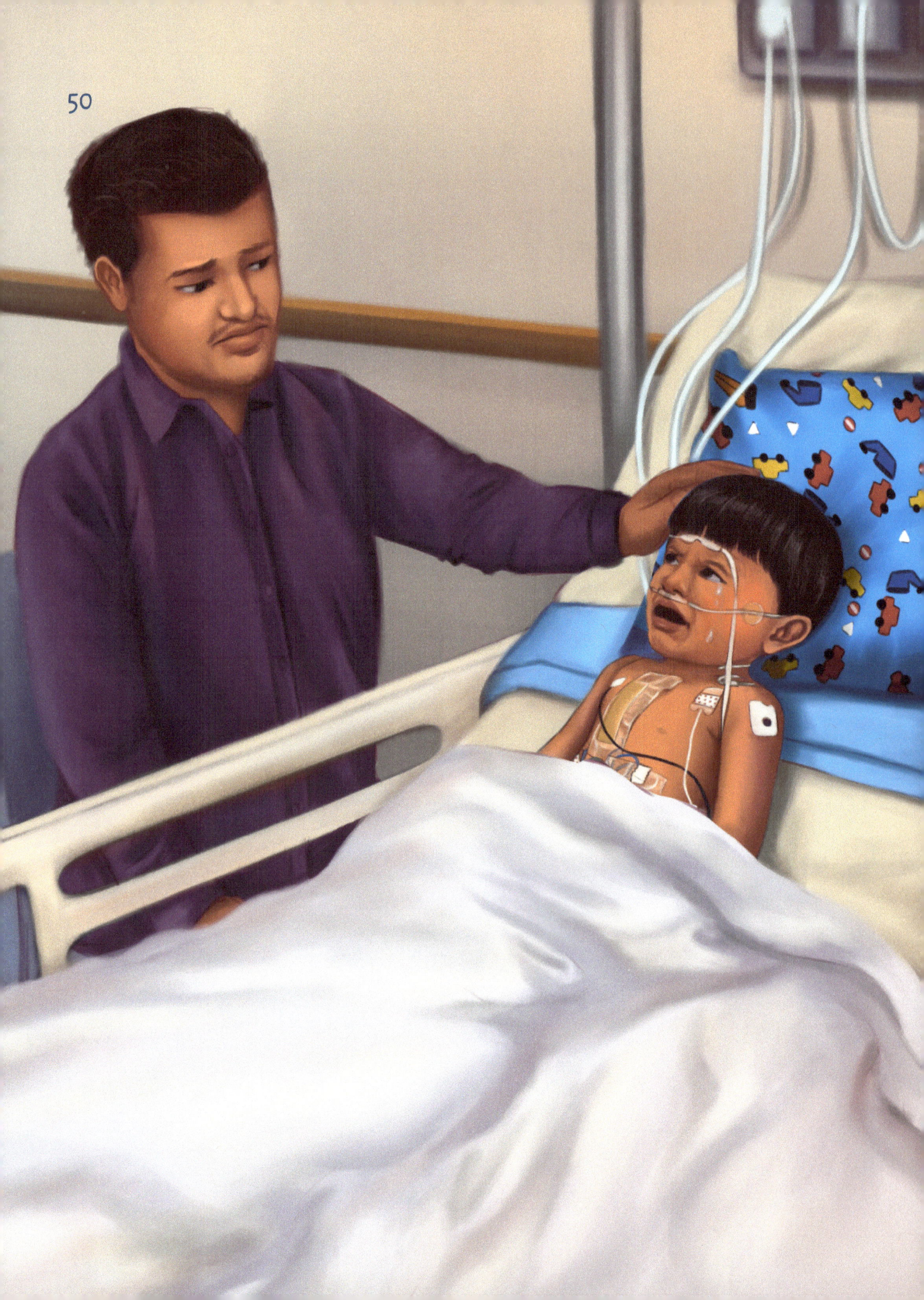

Boy's eyes open,

Mommy's here, thinking, words unspoken

Little boy's eyes look so glassy, broken

"I want my Mommy, I want my Daddy!" his first words shouted,

screaming, spoken!

Poor Boy's chest and body threaded with surgery tubes in...

Boy feels restless, anger, hunger, pain, and fear

He thinks out loud "OW! Why am I here?"

Mommy cries, "My precious dear," points to his chest

"because the doctor fixed you here."

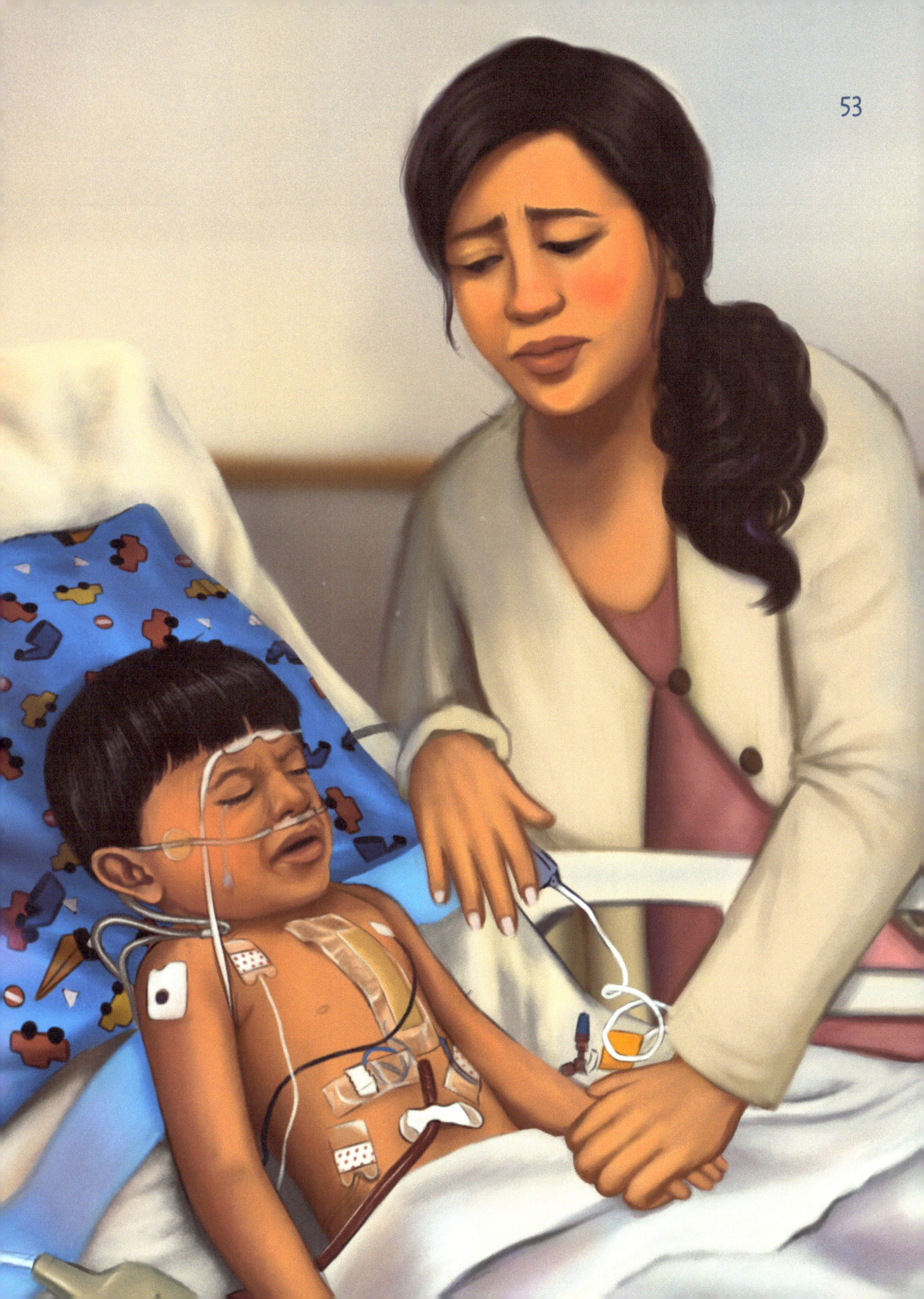

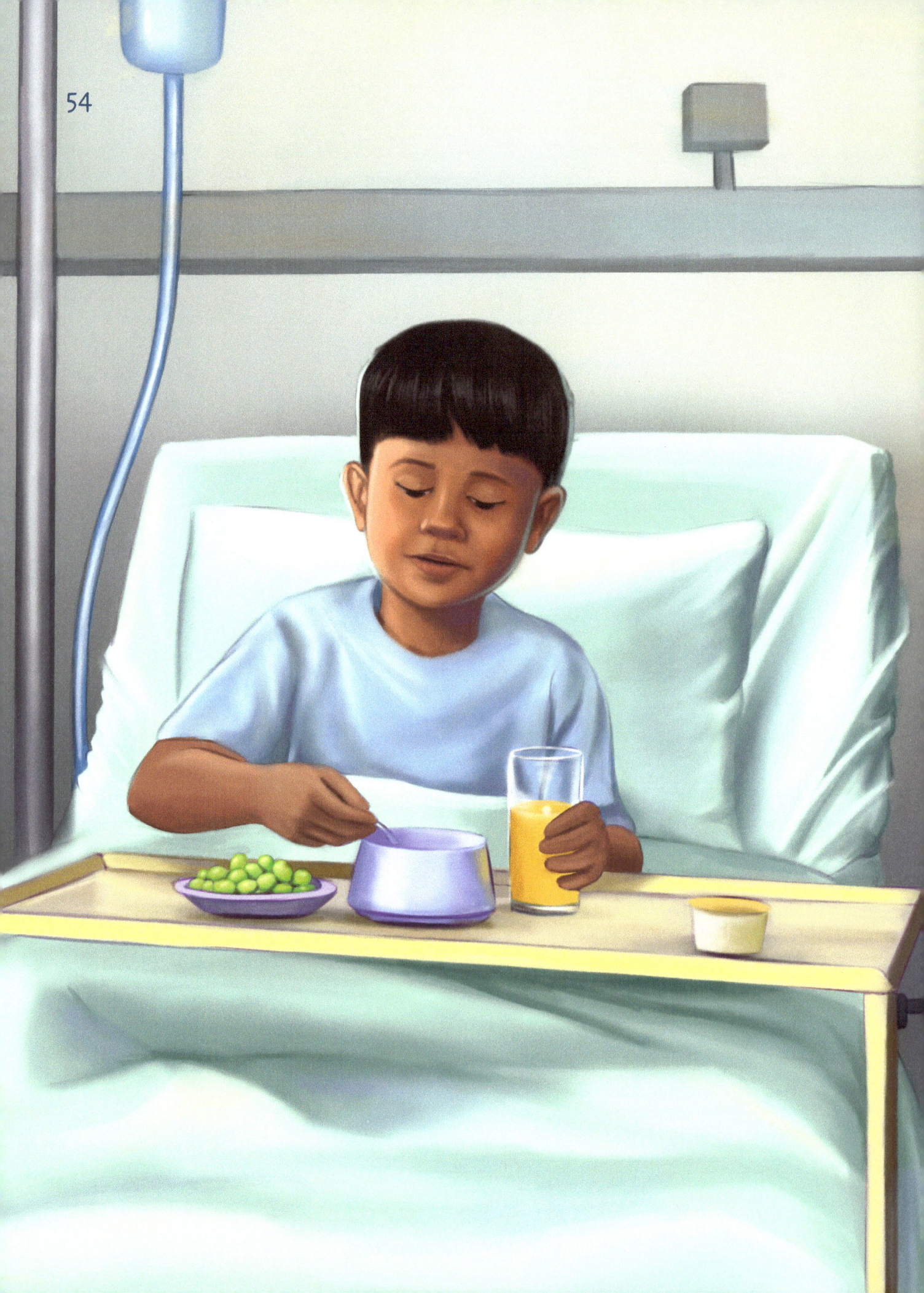

Little boy gets food and drink at last,

Surgery is over, now in the past,

He gets to moving really fast

X-rays, prods, pokes, another scan,

Walking faster, holding hands, riding hallway cars

just because he can,

Showing Mommy and Daddy that he is their strong little man

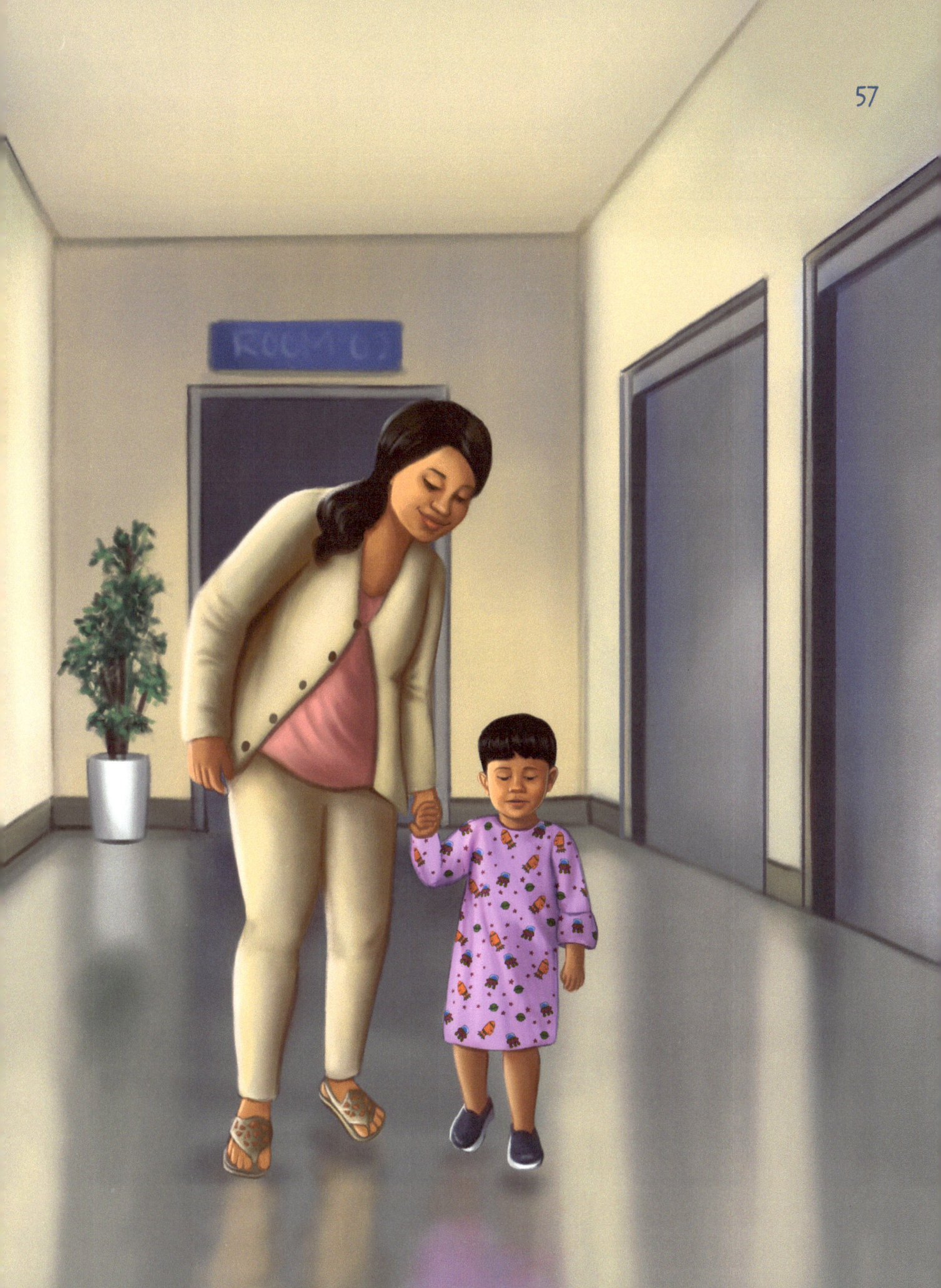

58

Doctors send him home at last

Surgery is over, now in the past

Baby, now a Boy is a DOUBLE Heart Warrior,

That coarc became inferior,

That atrial septal defect and mitral valve defect no longer superior,

Doctors, they stitched it up and closed it tight

Made it right,

At least for now, there'd be no more fright

But, BEWARE they warned, there is STILL no "cure"

These hazy visions are still obscure

Seated safely in the dark blue car,

the little Heart Warrior wears his tender, new, and healing scar,

heading home, which seems so far

Sister comes home,

and together they roam

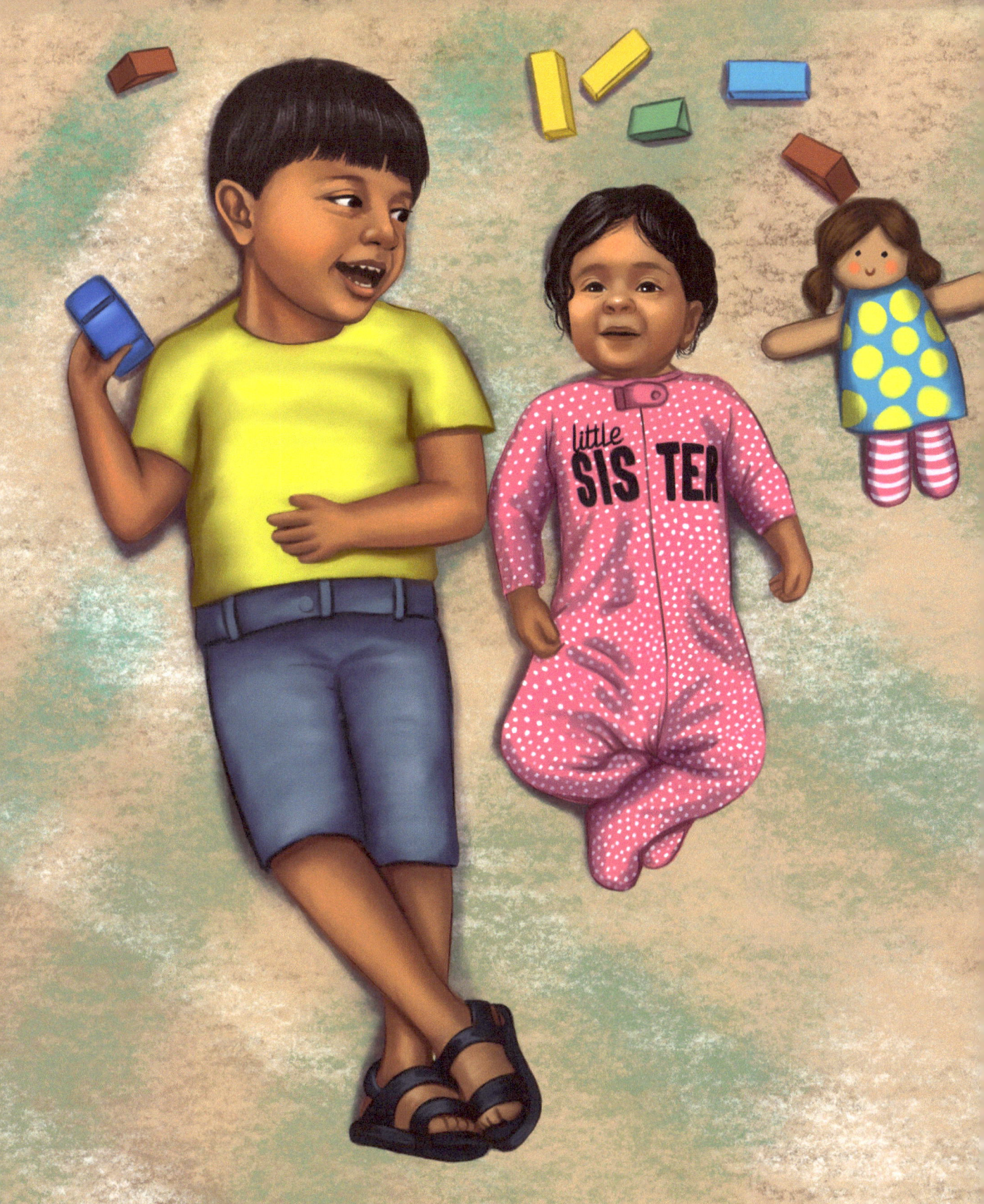

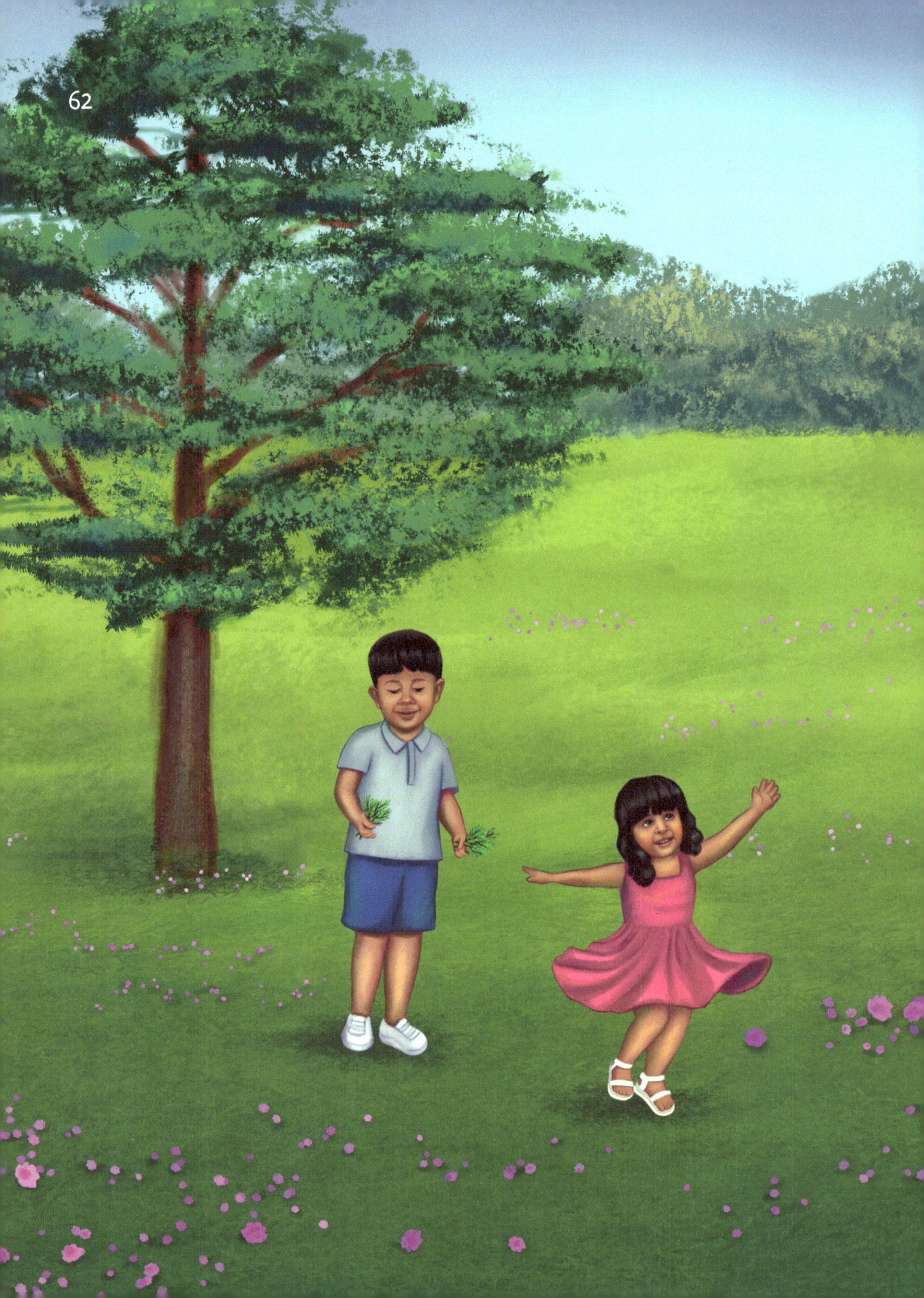

Thankful, grateful prayers to God on High

Looking way up into the sky,

Daddy, Mommy, Boy, and Sister cuddle, whisper, ponder why

and wish those surgery days GOOD BYE!

Sister's now quite the hip hop dancer,

and Heart Warrior Brother always the nature loving prancer

They learn together,

They grow together,

They love together

They fight together,

and THEY laugh TOGETHER

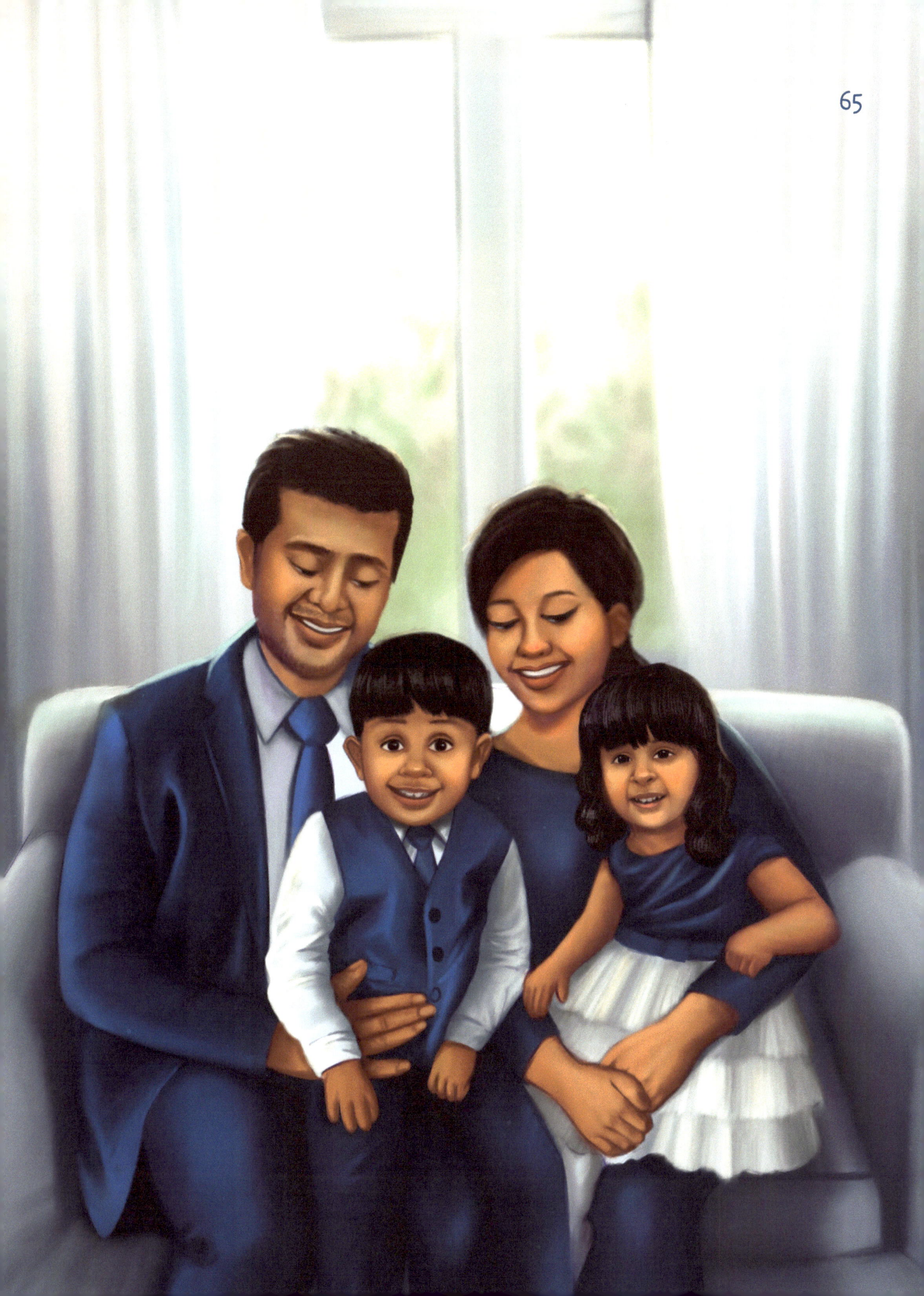

Acknowledgements

For my nature loving **heart**, **AuDHD**, and **7q.11.22** warrior, Elliot — this one is for you. May you continue to grow, rise up to challenges, and always be our shining star.

For Elliot's sister, Twyla — you will always be our intelligent, beautiful, strong, and brave princess. May you uphold your love, compassion, and devotion to your brother's care and growth.

For all the family, friends, and coworkers who have supported us during Elliot's surgeries.

For Dr. Fethke, Dr. MacMahon, and all the wonderful staff at Boston Children's Health Physicians who have worked so hard diagnosing and monitoring Elliot!

For Dr. Chen, Dr. Rome, all the nurses, techs, and other healthcare professionals at Children's Hospital of Philadelphia who gave our son his life back not once, but twice!

For Elliot's Preschool and Kindergarten teachers, aides, occupational, physical, and speech therapists; thank you for working with our little charmer and helping him to find the best in himself. He amazes us each and every day.

For our ever eternal, loving God, may you always look upon our family and help us to find the light in the tunnel when times are dark. You are always there for us.

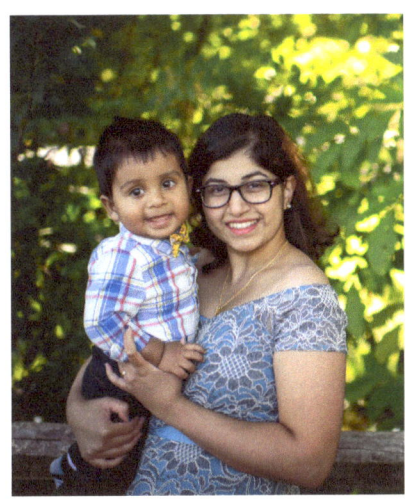

About the Author

Ashley K. George is a wife and mother of two kids; a Heart Warrior boy and a dancer girl. She enjoys writing poetry, children's books, and young adult books. She aims to spread her knowledge about disabilities, medical journeys, neurodiversity, and her culture. Ashley's previous books include *The Head in the Sky* and *Manju's Kerala Christmas*. She is also a New York and Maryland licensed Pediatric Speech Language Pathologist.

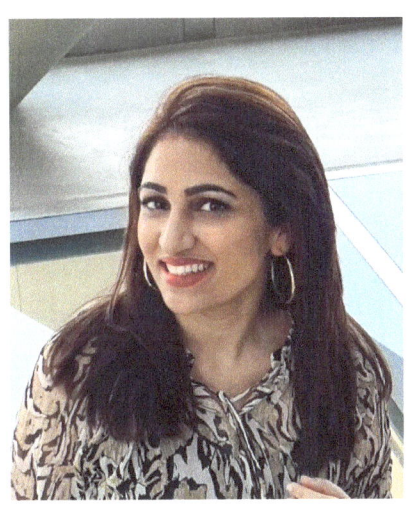

About the Illustrator

Sara Abbas is a Pakistani visual artist with an MFA in painting and drawing from Tulane University, New Orleans. Her illustration practice is centered around creating visuals for children's books in various art styles. She is currently working as a freelance illustrator and art instructor.

www.ingramcontent.com/pod-product-compliance
Lightning Source LLC
Chambersburg PA
CBHW040726060526
44119CB00083B/336